THE FORTRESS OF SOLITUDE

T.R. COCA

I0381959

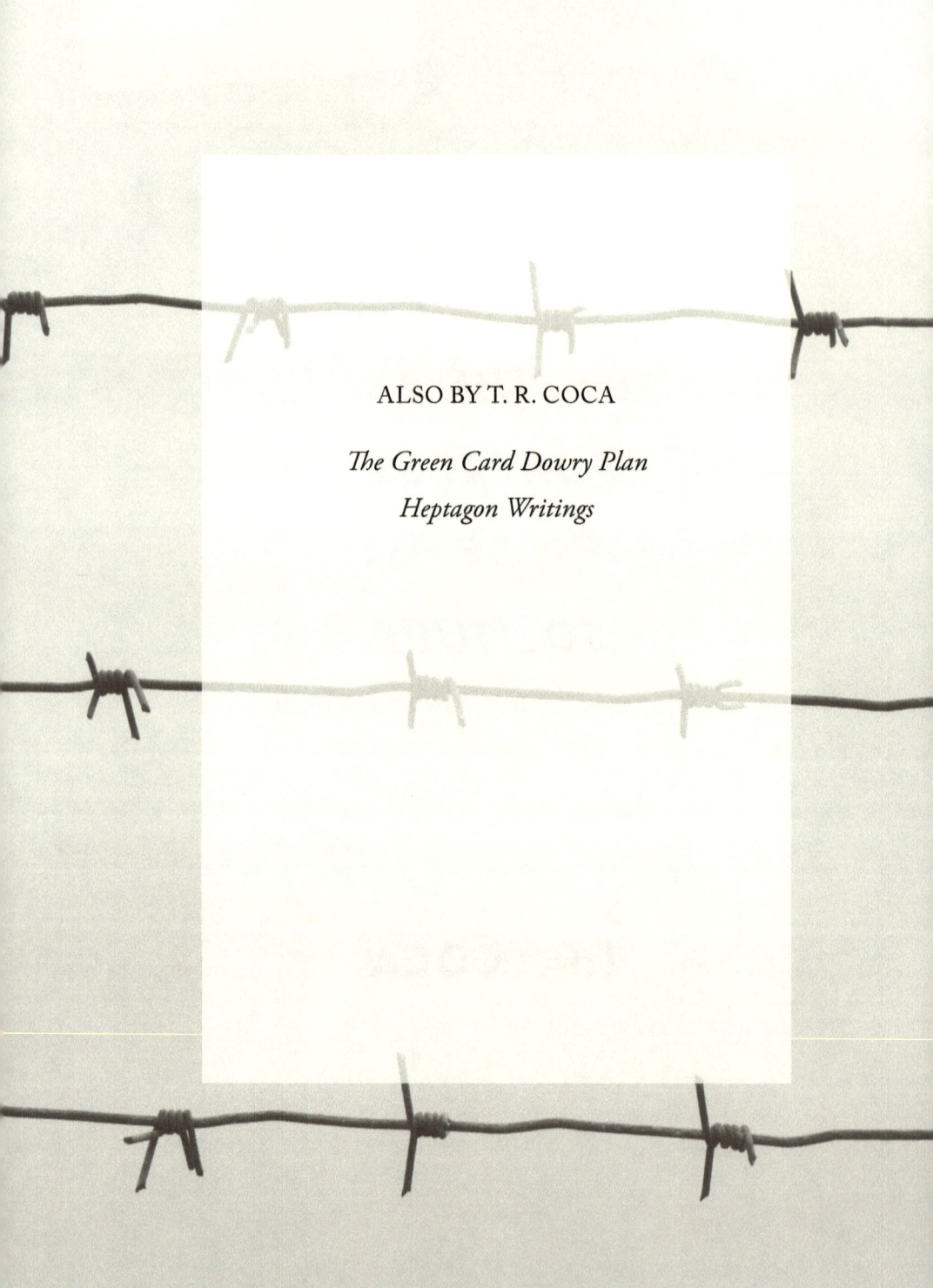

ALSO BY T. R. COCA

The Green Card Dowry Plan

Heptagon Writings

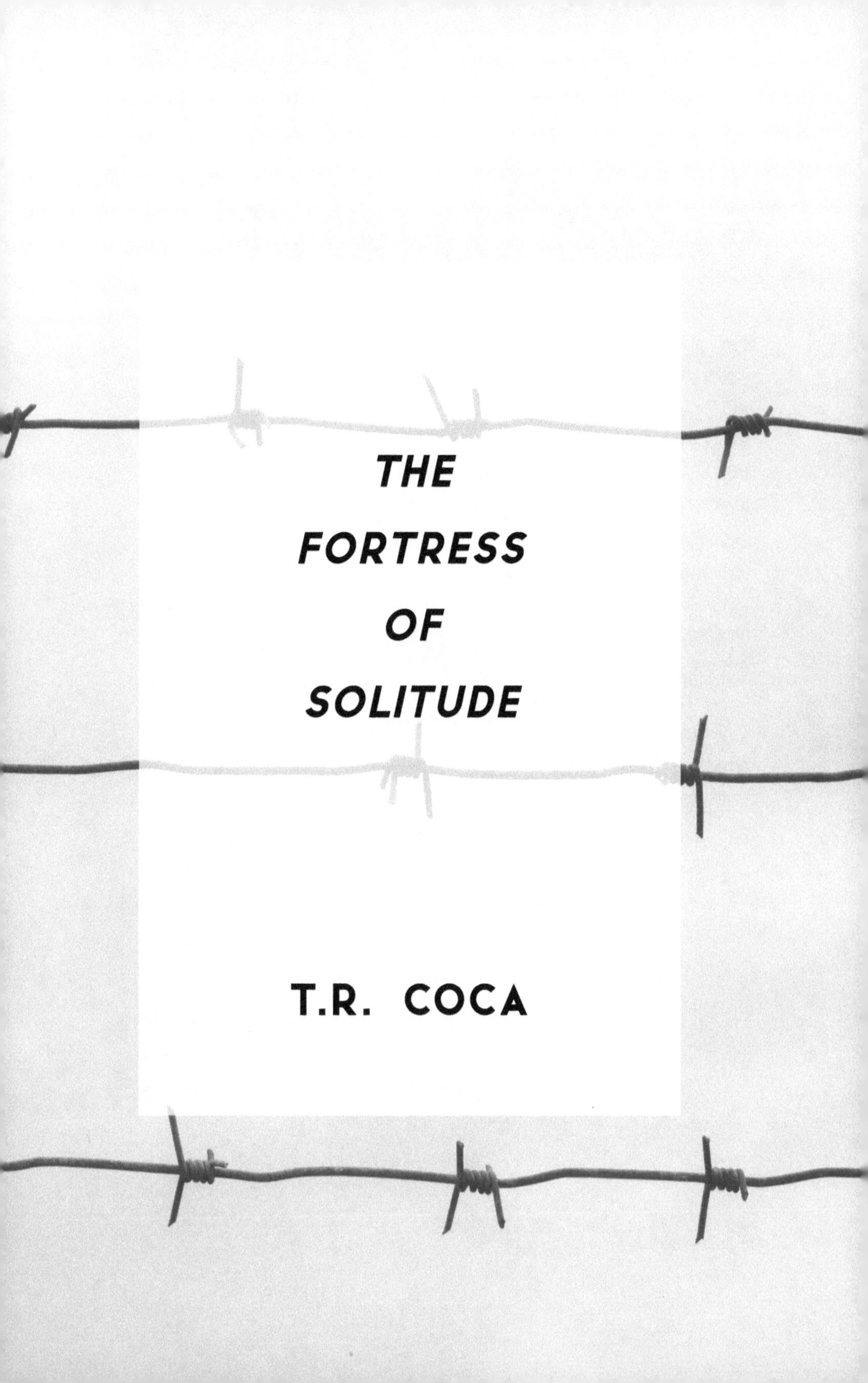

THE FORTRESS OF SOLITUDE

T.R. COCA

Copyright © 2021 by T.R. Coca

All rights reserved. No part of this publication may be reproduced, stored in a retrieval system, or transmitted in any form or by any means, electronic, mechanical, photocopying, recording, scanning, or otherwise, without the prior written permission of the author.

This is a work of pure imagination. None of the characters, businesses or institutions in this book is real. Specifically, the names, characters, businesses, institutions, places, events and incidents are products of author's fiction of imagination. Any resemblance to actual persons, living or dead or businesses, institutions and places is entirely coincidental.

Cover and interior design by The Book Cover Whisperer:
ProfessionalBookCoverDesign.com

ISBN: 978-1-7345338-5-9 Paperback
ISBN: 978-1-7345338-6-6 eBook

Printed in the United States of America

FIRST EDITION

CONTENTS

To my family – Rama and Dinesh

ABOUT THE STORY

It is a strange thing to think of the narrative of his life makes complete sense. He has been a strategist and planned his career and life with meticulous detail. Yet things somehow have gone wrong.

With disturbing anecdotes, the arranged marriage of a romantic couple's wishes pulls them in different directions. What happens when a spouse goes rogue with malice aforethought and unfairly humiliates and punishes the other and connives to embrace an old flame.

Retribution? But at what cost?

Imaginative and engaging characters weave genuine outrages of human venality.

Suspense and fascination unravels when the elite corps of the Secret Service, FBI, National Security Agency and ICE prosecutes a threat against a high level elected government official transforming his life into a taut and chilling drama.

His life story is full of international intrigue with an unpredictable ending when a cold-blooded and ruthless hired killer gets involved.

CHAPTER

1

IT WAS A COLD MORNING in the fall. The air in mid-November was crisp. Ashwin Sharma awoke before sunrise in his apartment in Providence, Rhode Island. He thought of going back to catch more sleep, but the thoughts in his head kept him from taking more naps. As the traces of dawn peaked through the French door in his bedroom leading to a balcony, he concluded that he had too many activities planned for the day to sleep more.

After all today is going to be the last day of his stay in America since he decided to leave the country and go back home. He wanted to honor the legal constraint imposed on him by the U.S. Immigration & Naturalization Service.

He will hand over the keys to his apartment to his landlord and officially vacate the place which he essentially completed the previous day by selling off most of his personal possessions. The only possessions he is now left with are a suitcase which he filled with his clothes and memorabilia, a hand-carry luggage where he stored his more valuable clothes and a backpack which contained his laptop, a cell phone, passport and other essential items he needed for traveling.

Ash woke up, brushed his teeth, got a clean shave and showered before he walked over to the bakery in the next block to his apartment building. He ordered a buttery croissant which he loved and a cup of piping hot and strong coffee. It was a perfect breakfast which he enjoyed in quiet solitude at one of the open tables inside the warm bakery filled with sweet cinnamon in the air.

He waited for the branch of the Bank of America to open at 9 O' clock. He had checking and savings accounts in that bank. He walked over to the bank two blocks away around 9 AM, approached as the first customer of an open teller.

"Hello, I have two accounts here. I would like to close them," he announced.

The teller, who was a pretty blond with long hair and in her early twenties, curiously asked, "Why do you wish to close your accounts with our bank?"

Ash replied, "I am leaving the country today. There is no reason to keep my accounts open any longer."

The teller complied with his request. She handed him two withdrawal slips and asked him to fill out and also write his forwarding address.

He filled out the slips one for each of his accounts and withdrew all the balance of over four thousand and thirty seven dollars he saved. The teller counted forty crisp one-hundred dollar currency bills and the additional amount in small bills as he attentively looked at her counting. He tucked the currency in his bulging wallet and left the bank and headed back to his apartment.

As scheduled, the landlord showed up at his apartment at 10 O' clock. Ash and the landlord went through his small and cleaned up apartment for the final inspection of its condition. Ash has always been fastidious. He kept his place immaculate, almost obsessively clean.

The landlord was satisfied with the condition of the premises and filled out a form which proclaimed that the unit was in satisfactory condition. That form released Ash from liability for any damage to the unit. Ash provided his overseas address for the landlord to mail the security deposit he paid months earlier when he leased the unit under a short-term rental agreement.

It was 11 AM now. Ash had ample time to drive the Hertz rental car which he leased the previous night to drive to Newark International airport in New Jersey to catch his flight overseas.

Ash booked a one-way ticket on United Airlines for a non-stop flight from Newark to the Indira Gandhi International airport in New Delhi. He booked a premium economy class seat. United notified him the previous day that Ash was upgraded to the business class. Ash put in many miles on United in his previous travels both domestically and internationally and accumulated sufficient loyalty to garner his present upgrade.

Ash was in no hurry to drive to Newark as he had plenty of time to catch his scheduled flight. The flight was scheduled to depart Newark airport at 9:07 PM and arrive in New Delhi at 9:05 the next evening after a long nonstop flight of nearly fourteen hours.

Ash's final destination is Hyderabad in southern Indian state of Andhra Pradesh. That is where his mother and father live now and that is where he grew up until he arrived in the U.S. seven years ago. He is booked on Jet Air for a flight from New Delhi to Hyderabad on the morning after the United Airlines flight landed in the nation's capital.

—

TODAY IS THE LAST DAY of his stay in the United States. "*God knows when I will be back again,*" Ash said to himself. He decided to take a drive to see the fall foliage in the Hudson Valley in the New York state which he visited once before.

So instead of heading southwest along the Atlantic coast on interstate 95, he headed directly west across Connecticut to catch interstate 84. This highway took him toward the Hudson River in New York State with the mountainous terrain and tree-lined highways and rural farmlands of the Putnam and Duchess Counties. He drove into the town of Beacon perched along the Hudson River at around 2 PM.

Beacon reached the peak foliage with more than eighty percent color change and with a more significant color along the banks of the Hudson River and the surrounding hills and nearby mountains. Bright yellow, red, orange and purple leaves glistened in the bright sun light filling the sight with spectacular autumn hues. Rust was forming on some red maple leaves. "*Oh! God! What a beautiful day!*" Ash said to himself at the palette of mid-autumn he was witnessing as he drove.

Ash decided to stop for lunch as he smelled the whiff of the fresh meat of tasty burgers being cooked on an open-air charcoal grill. He pulled over at the Hudson House on the Main Street of Cold Spring which offered outdoor seating overlooking the Hudson. This was a gem of a restaurant which he visited years before. The waiter showed him a lovely spot on the deck with a beautiful view of the riverfront across the street. He ordered a Black Angus burger and sweet potato fries. The burger was appetizingly huge, juicy and cooked perfectly to his liking. He took a bite of the served burger. The special sauce from the burger oozed into his fingers. He could only finish half of the delicious burger.

He slipped into his car and headed east toward the Bear Mountain State Parkway driving through Peekskill to access the southbound Taconic Parkway. He loved driving along the Taconic's winding highway with stone retaining walls and a canopy of trees. The season offered spectacular and vivid colors of the Canadian maples. The southern end the Taconic Parkway led him to the Saw Mill River Parkway in West Chester County. Ash crossed the Hudson at the George Washington Bridge into New Jersey and headed south to Newark International Airport.

—

Ash returned the rental car and checked in at the United Airlines ticket counter in Newark International. It was almost 6 PM. He checked in his large suitcase and completed his passport check and went through the TSA checkpoint for airport security. Ash found his way to the Red Carpet lounge to hang out before boarding commenced.

Boarding of United flight 801 from Newark to New Delhi was called by the lounge hostess at 7:40 PM. Ash tossed his backpack on his shoulder rolled his hand-carry and headed to the boarding gate.

As he embarked the plane, he noticed that the economy class appeared full. The business class was not full.

A female flight attendant greeted him with a shiny white smile radiating from her teeth as he entered the business class cabin. She looked at his boarding pass and showed him his assigned window seat 8A. He glanced at his leathery-lined seat which invited him for a comfortable accommodation. He stowed his hand-carry bag in the overhead compartment above his seat and settled into 8A by throwing his back-pack under the seat in front of him.

Soon another charming flight attendant brought him a tray containing a choice of small tumblers filled with orange juice, cold water, and short-stemmed glasses of red and white wines and bubbling flutes of Champagne and offered to him. Ash picked up the Champagne and sipped. Seat 8B next to him remained unoccupied.

Ash pulled the Hemisphere's magazine from the front seat pocket and thumbed through it for interesting articles. An article titled "Honeymoon in Maldives" caught his attention. He had never been to Maldives. He wished he spent his honeymoon on these tranquil islands in the Indian Ocean. Instead, his honeymoon was spent in Srinagar, Kashmir where the perennial clashes between the Indian and Pakistani separatists kept the honeymoon couple on their toes on their last day and robbed them of the peace and tranquility they hoped to enjoy.

More Champagne refilled his flute as the flight attendant moved around the cabin to see who needed more drinks. On-time departure passed. The plane continued to be held at the gate. Minutes ticked by.

Finally, the captain came on the passenger address system and explained to the passengers the reason for the delay, "Thunderstorms across the northeastern parts of the United States and the Canadian provinces are holding up our on-time departure. We would be here perhaps half-an-hour for the storms to pass."

Ash believed what the captain stated. All that was holding up the plane's departure was the weather.

The flight attendant who was attending to him was busy at work. She brought more cabin drinks and this time brought him mixed nuts warmed in the oven. Ash glanced out of the plane's tiny window. The activity on the ground below and around the aircraft appeared normal. The main cabin door remained open as if to take on more passengers. The jet bridge was still in its place and no instruction was forthcoming from the captain for the cabin to be prepared for takeoff.

Ash was lost in his thoughts as he sipped the Champagne and munched the warm nuts and gazed the sky from his airplane window.

Just then a man's voice from the aisle of his row spoke, "Sir, are you Mr. Sharma. Ashwin Sharma?" he queried.

Ash turned to the man. Two other burly men were standing next to him in the aisle area. One of the men carried a United Airlines gold badge affixed to his jacket. He looked like a United's Security officer. The other two who wore blue suits didn't have identification badges on their lapels.

Ash answered, "Yes, I am, Ashwin Sharma."

"Mr. Sharma, could you come with us please," the same man politely asked. The man paused and continued, "We are the Special Agents of the FBI. We need to have a talk off the airplane."

Ash inquisitively and politely asked, "What is the reason, Sir?"

"Please simple come with us. We have a few questions to ask," was the man's reply.

Ash had no choice with the three burly men standing in the aisle and confronting him. Ash asked, "Can I leave my belongings on the plane?"

The reply to his query was stern, "No. Please collect your belongings. We do not wish to hold up the plane any longer from its scheduled departure time which I believe has already passed," and looked at the United's Security Officer next to him who nodded in agreement.

Ash then realized that he is being ejected from the plane. He could have resisted but realized that he will cause a scene and the burly men would force him out of the plane and may handcuff him.

Ash picked up his backpack and was about to reach the overhead compartment to access his carry-on suitcase. Just then the United Officer grabbed the carry-on. Ash followed the FBI agents with the United Security Officer wheeling his carry-on luggage behind the agents.

CHAPTER

2

ASHWIN SHARMA LED AN UNEVENTFUL life for the most part. He was born into a middle class, well-to-do Hindu family in India. His father Sunil Sharma was employed as an Officer with the Indian Customs Agency which position, he earned after completing his Indian Administrative Services examination. He has been living in Hyderabad all of his life. He has been placed at the Rajiv Gandhi International Airport in Hyderabad to monitor possible Indian Custom's law violations by the arriving and departing international passengers.

Ash' mother Rupa Sharma was an educated stay-at-home mother of two sons: he and his brother Samir who was five years older than him. Education and studiousness were emphasized by Ash's parents. His father pushed both sons to major in physical sciences, particularly physics, technology, engineering and mathematics, which they pursued wholeheartedly.

Ash is smart and organized. He loved chess as a child. He played it at school and at home with his brother and father. He was good at it. It taught him logic and developed his mind to think strategically. Ash had more capacity for left brain thinking from childhood. Chess is highly analytical and enabled him to focus accurately on a problem and think many steps ahead before he made a move.

Ash had a normal childhood. His parents accepted him for who he was. They did not have preset expectation to fulfill their dreams and did not try to mold him or his brother into some one different than they actually were. His parents helped Ash to tolerate frustration by not giving everything that he wanted, but also by not depriving him of everything he wanted. That helped Ash to build good ego strength early in his life which would come handy later in his life.

Having developed an analytical mind, Ash earned excellent education in high school which enabled him to attend the top-ranking engineering college in Hyderabad, the Indian Institute of Technology -Hyderabad. The IIT-Hyderabad, as it was called for brevity, had just opened its brand-new campus.

It was a modern facility with ultra-modern infrastructure from classrooms to sports grounds. Everything was well maintained and the institution was located in a park-like setting.

Because of the excellent grades Ash earned before IIT-Hyderabad, he managed to receive a fifty thousand rupee exemption toward his annual tuition, which was a great help to his father as it took care of a significant portion of the tuition costs. As was expected, Ash stayed with his parents white attending the IIT-Hyderabad.

As part of the elected curriculum for completing his degree of

Bachelor of Technology he took advanced courses in computer network software architecture and mobile communication software. IIT-Hyderabad placed him with Microsoft (India) which is a wholly owned subsidiary of the Microsoft Corporation headquartered in the U.S.

Dubbed as the HITECH City, Microsoft India Development Center was one of the early U.S. tech companies to open in this City on the outskirts of Hyderabad. Microsoft housed a research and development campus where open labs and state-of-the-art innovation space were used to advance various software projects that the company was championing.

Microsoft just then acquired Nokia's handset business by spending nearly $8 billion to compete with Apple's iOS and Google's Android operating systems used in their mobile cell phone businesses. Ash was assigned a project to work on Windows-based communication software that Nokia was previously developing. This project actually drove Microsoft's acquisition of the handset business from Nokia.

Ash enjoyed working at Microsoft although the HITECH City was located twenty miles away from home. He was forced to take two buses and spend over an hour each way to get to and return from work every day. He detested the long commute which became more miserable during the monsoon season.

His immediate manager at Microsoft and his colleagues were amiable and were good to collaborate and work on many exciting projects that the headquarters in Redmond, Washington passed on to his team. Ash participated in frequent voice and video conferences with project leaders in Redmond who steered him to compete in a race between the Indian team and the headquarters' team for successful integration of the Windows operating system software with the Nokia handsets.

Ash's brother Sunil was already in the U.S. He is also specialized in computer sciences. Having left India three or four years earlier, he has been employed with Fidelity Investments in Raleigh, North Carolina.

—

ASH'S PARENTS ENCOURAGED their sons to take risks and were ready to help them with their personal difficulties. They expected Ash to follow his brother's footsteps and go to the U.S. Their expectation was that both sons would gain valuable experience by working in America. They also expected that their sons one day will return to India after earning money and establish themselves close to home.

Ash figured out that the easiest way to find employment in the U.S. is through the H1B visa program which provides permits by the U.S. government for a limited number of foreigners to work for a U.S.-based employer. The conditions for the H1B visa were that the foreign worker must have a graduate level university degree and is qualified to work in a specialized field that the employer was unable to fill from a U.S.-based work pool.

Ash found himself in an idyllic situation where he stood a good chance to be sponsored by Microsoft for the coveted H1B visa. He is a graduate of IIT, which is a top-rated educational institution. He has already worked on a special project with Microsoft where the integration of the newly acquired handset business with the Windows operating system software is critical. Ash realized that he stood an excellent chance to qualify for the H1B permit.

Being a strategic thinker Ash figured out that by being employed at Microsoft in Hyderabad he needed to have a manager in Microsoft's headquarters to sponsor him for his H1B visa with the U.S. Customs & Immigration Services.

He drew up a long-term plan to permanently immigrate to the U.S. Once he reached the U.S. under the H1B visa it is good for three years; and if needed it can be extended up to six years. If he performed well for Microsoft then his boss in Redmond would file the paperwork with USCIS to facilitate a change of immigration status from the H1B to permanent residency, known as the green card. Earning the green card is his ultimate goal.

—

Ash was in no rush to pull the trigger on his H1B work permit by Microsoft. He enjoyed his life as a bachelor but did not date any girls as his parents did not favor such socializing with girls. He enjoyed going the Bollywood movies, listening to lively Hindi music and dining in high class restaurants which catered the Indian food. He loved eating the Mysore masala *dosa* for lunch and the Hyderabadi mutton biriyani for dinner. He craved for spicy meals with locally brewed fine beers which ameliorated the sting of the spicy food in his mouth as he feasted.

Despite the limitations on socializing with girls, a fellow member in his team by the name of Malini caught Ash's attention. Mal, as she wanted to be addressed, worked as a project administrator for the cloud computing platform that Microsoft began to heavily invest in developing to compete with IBM and Amazon. Mal's job was to prepare documentation and project plans for the platform she was assigned. She and Ash reported to the same manager and participated in group meetings and were generally familiar with each other at a professional level.

Mal was tall and slender with nut-brown hair and soft-skinned appearance, particularly a smooth face. With an innocent face, she presented the appearance of a sixteen- or seventeen-year-old girl.

It was the aura of innocence and trustworthiness she carried that put Ash at ease and drew his attraction to her.

Ash wanted to find out more about Mal's thoughts on career and what her life's desires were. On a rainy monsoon evening Mal had to work late because the manager wanted all the documents to be made ready for delivery the next morning. All of the employees left for the evening. Only the manager and Mal were working frantically to get the documents gathered. Ash took pity on his colleague as she was scrambling to get the documents printed and stack them into neat piles.

Ask decided that he would stay back not only because he detested traveling in the rain, but took pity on Mal. He wanted to extend a helping hand or else provide moral support for her hard work. Finally the project work was done around ten O'clock. Mal thanked Ash for staying late and helping her out.

It was late for the city buses to run at that hour. Ash called for a taxi. They sat on the back seat and did not engage much in conversation. Rain flew horizontally and lashed the windshield of the taxi.

Mal pulled a small cotton kerchief from her purse. It was laced with a lavender scent which immediately pervaded the space in the small taxi. The taxi driver muttered, "Smells good." The soggy air quickly dissipated the burst of fragrance.

For forty five minutes they rode the taxi silently gazing out of the taxi windows. Neither of them engaged even in small talk as the taxi driver understood English and the couple did not want him to listen to their conversation. Ash asked the taxi driver to drop Mal off at her house on Majid Road first and then asked to continue the drive to his house.

—

A MONTH LATER ON A Saturday Ash went to work to finish up some unfinished work. He was bored of working. He decided to call Mal at home and engaged in a personal conversation. While talking, Ash wanted to find out whether Mal has any romantic feelings toward him. He decided to play a little innocent game with her when she asked, "Ash, what are you planning to do after you completed the handset project?"

Ash quickly replied, "I am planning to leave the company."

Mal questioned him with great surprise, "What! Why do you want to leave Microsoft?"

Ash replied "I always wanted to work in Bengaluru. Perhaps, IBM in Bengaluru would be a good place to work for. IBM is a software powerhouse in cloud computing, you know?"

Mal felt disappointed. She drew in a long breath and commented, "I think it is reasonable for you to try working at another multinational company to diversify your career path and expand your network of connections."

She continued, "Ash, you know you are a good employee and I watched you in our team. You were always focused and it would be great loss if you were to leave Microsoft."

Toward the end of their conversation Mal sounded heavy. Ash could feel that she was about to cry. He asked, "Mal, are you saddened by my decision?"

Mal broke down and started crying as if in despair.

Ash asked, "Why are you crying?"

Mal admitted "I like you Ash. I was hoping we would be able to date."

Mal added, "It would be devastating for me that you would move away. We would not have time to date and get to know each other."

Ash was pleasantly surprised by her secret intention to date him.

Ash immediately apologized for the prank he played on her. He conceded, "Mal, I am going nowhere. Please be assured that leaving Microsoft was just a random thought. I love my job at Microsoft and plan to remain here."

With this exchange concluded to Mal's great relief, the two started dating the Indian way, hiding from her parents and sneaky meet ups.

Ash, however, informed his parents about the sweet girl Mal from his office that he is dating. His parents were perfectly okay with it.

As Mal and Ash got serious about being with each other so much so that she was agreeable to address her as Malli, which meant the fragrant flower of white jasmine in her mother tongue. It was time to meet her dad.

Mal's father was a serious man. Gruff in the voice he spoke and a bit stressed which showed on his wrinkled face. He was short, five feet in height. He was pudgy. They sat on airy wicker chairs in the veranda of his house.

One of the serious first questions he asked Ash was, "What are your future plans Ashwin?"

Ash responded politely, "I am not sure. I started working at Microsoft only recently and have no idea what I wanted to do in the long run." Ash did not want to share his plans which he already laid out which was to work in the U.S. for a while and then return to India and settle down.

Ash wanted to know where Mal's dad was leading to and what his expectations were.

Mal's father asked, "Do you have any desire to move to America?"

Ash demurred by hanging his head down.

Ash's silence was construed by her dad that Ash is not a potential candidate for an alliance with Mal.

Her father made clear of his expectations of a suitor for his daughter by saying, "My daughter would marry only a guy who has serious plans to move to America. I prefer a bachelor who is already settled in America to marry her. That makes it easy for Mal to immigrate to the U.S. and settle down and establish her family there."

Ash became somewhat uncomfortable with that remark. His discomfort grew somewhat into a mild fury. Ash did not like the idea his daughter should marry a guy who is settled in the U.S. With that Ash, without displaying his anger, politely walked out of his house, bidding the family good bye.

Ash did not break up with Mal right away. He waited until her dad finalized a guy who was already working in the U.S. to wed his daughter. During that period Ash's life was turned upside down as he liked Mal's sweet and kind nature. He thought that they made a compatible couple. However, Mal's nature was to be subservient to her father's wishes.

After the arranged marriage of Mal was finalized it was no fun for Ash to meet her as they reached a dead-end in their relationship. Soon Mal got married and she was gone.

The short romantic affair with Mal only made Ash in a weird way to be more determined to go to the U.S. It dawned on him that carrying a U.S. residential address enhanced his opportunities of finding a suitable marriage partner from India. Nevertheless, Ash stuck to his original strategy to go to the U.S. when the time was ripe for him.

—

Two years passed by as Ash delved more and more into the specialized software for the handsets he was developing at Microsoft. He was invited to a face-to-face meeting in Redmond; purportedly to discuss the complexities of the adaptation of the Windows software for the Nokia cell phone.

He traveled on a visitor's visa to Redmond. That was his first visit to the U.S. He was excited.

He just fell in love with Microsoft's campus at the headquarters in Redmond. It was serene place where thousands of employees, including some who were born in India, worked. All the employees he met on his short visit were focused on their jobs and seemed highly educated in engineering, computer architecture; and some majored in humanities which somewhat surprised Ash because they were working with engineers in the aesthetic aspects of the design of Microsoft's hardware.

On this visit to Microsoft's head office one manager Nicola Erwasti took a special interest in Ash's work. Erwasti himself transitioned to the headquarters from his previous job at Nokia in Espoo in Finland because of Microsoft's acquisition of the Finnish icon. He was very impressed with Ash' deep knowledge of the problems he was confronting to adapt the Windows operating system software to the Nokia handsets. He closely monitored Ash while he plowed through the software he was asked to handle from Hyderabad.

Erwasti advised Ash to keep him informed in real time of the progress he was making after he returned home. Ash felt good that he made a positive impression on Erwasti, which is the outcome he planned for his short visit.

Sure enough after Ash returned home to Hyderabad, his manager invited him to his office and posed this question, "Ash, you have been doing commendable work on the handsets. The headquarters is impressed as well. They would like you to move to Redmond on a short term basis. Are you interested?"

Ash could hardly conceal his merriment at the offer. He quietly replied, "Sure. I loved the campus at the headquarters in my last visit. However, let me ask for your guidance."

"Do you see a downside to my going to America?" Ash asked.

The manger replied, "Ash, this is an once-in-a-lifetime opportunity. Many of your colleagues would kill for such an opportunity. I see only positive attributes to this expressed interest by the headquarters."

"If I were to accept, who would I be working for at the headquarters?" Ash queried.

The manager replied, "Most probably, you will team with the group headed by Nicola Erwasti." He continued, "You met Erwasti on your last trip. Didn't you?"

Ash nodded in the affirmative.

Ash asked him for the timeline of his assignment. He was told, "As soon as the paperwork is completed, probably in about a month or six weeks."

Ash replied, "Yes, I am interested in this U.S. assignment, but I need to check with my parents, too."

With those words uttered, Ash left the meeting. He was gleeful. He congratulated himself that his laid-out plan is on track.

Leaving his parents and his comfortable home where everything was provided for and starting a new life in a foreign country appeared overwhelming to Ash. The fact that his brother was already there, albeit three time zones away and separated by over two thousand miles, gave Ash some comfort.

After a couple of days of back and forth with his manager, Ash notified him that he decided to try out the assignment in the U.S. However, he kept the offer a secret and decided to tell his family and friends after he received the H1B visa.

—

Within two months Mr. Erwasti through the Human Resources Department in Microsoft, Redmond petitioned Ash for a H1B visa which was readily approved by USCIS. The approved documents were delivered to Ash to have him fetch his temporary work permit from the U.S. Consulate in Hyderabad.

The interview with the Consulate was perfunctory as Ash graduated from a highly reputed college in India and the offer letter and other supporting documents came from a well-known multinational company. Ash merely had to produce his Indian passport and the documents he received from his employer.

The Consulate General greeted Ash, asked a few simple questions and perused the documents Ash produced. Within an hour Ash's name was called by the visa counter at the Consulate. Ash picked up the H1B visa and left the Consulate.

Ash was excited that he successfully completed a key phase in his well-laid out journey to go to the United Sates to work. At the same time, he was a bit scared.

He celebrated his H1B visa grant by having a beer bash with his friends followed by a sumptuous dinner at the Taj hotel. The following week he was off to Seattle-Tacoma International airport in the state of Washington to start his assignment at Microsoft's headquarters in nearby Redmond.

—

With more than forty-five thousand employees the Microsoft

headquarters impressed Ash even more than his first visit months earlier. He quickly found an apartment to share at a location dubbed as The Campus.

The Campus had a medley of restaurants and shops and with car-free pedestrian zones. Shuttles arranged by Microsoft took him from The Campus to his place of work at the headquarters and he did not immediately need a car to get around.

Ash shared his two-bedroom apartment with Mann Singh who worked on the next generation of the X-Box console. Mann was from Gurgaon near New Delhi.

He had been with Microsoft for over five years. He wore a colorful turban around his head and face each day and was outgoing with everyone on The Campus. Like Ash, Mann loved Bollywood movies. He was an entertainer and drew crowds when he played music on his boom box and engaged in the rhythmic bhangra dance with girls on The Campus.

What attracted Ash the most at the headquarters were the large number of Indian restaurants sprinkled throughout Redmond and Seattle. He loved frequenting with Singh and other friends he made the Mayuri Indian Cuisine restaurant near The Campus which offered excellent northern and southern India classics as well as a vegetarian menu.

—

It was a balmy day in Redmond. It stopped drizzling incessantly for seven days. The humidity was below normal for the Seattle area that day. Ash and Mann Singh sat at a park bench on park-like and manicured grounds of The Campus as they watched people mulling around. A young couple was walking their dog. Others were scurrying on their activities.

The previous day Ash indulged in a self-guided tour through the doors of the Microsoft Visitor Center. He was impressed by the many innovations and exciting technologies that were created by the company which were on display at the Center. That visit sparked more interest in Ash to understand Microsoft's corporate history.

Singh knew about the history of Microsoft's executive management. Ash took the opportunity and asked him, "Mann, could you share with me what you know about the recent history of the company's upper management? You have been with his company for a while. I would like to be educated on this history."

Singh obliged, "Ash, you should understand that Microsoft's management at the corporate level has been trudging through an unprecedented transformation. A few years ago the founder Bill Gates, after running the company for twenty five years, handed the reins to his co-founder Steve Ballmer. Despite Ballmer's remarkable financial performance of over a billion dollars of profit month after month the company's stock price did not advance up. Microsoft ceded its market share in the search business to Google and in the smartphone business to Apple."

Singh continued his discourse, "The shares of Microsoft languished in the range of twenty to thirty dollars per share for years. The shareholders, especially large institutional shareholders, agitated Bill Gates and Ballmer to bring changes to the business and make the stock price grow.

"Ballmer, who regularly played competitive basketball after work with his coworkers on Microsoft's courts, then decided to play hardball with Apple in the smartphone business. He plunked nearly $8 billion to purchase the handset business from Nokia, which had a remarkable market share selling its cell phones. Ballmer believed that he would kill two birds in one shot. He would dethrone Apple in its iPhone sales; and vigorously compete with the newly emerging Google which uses the Android operating system in its phones" Singh said.

Ash then piped in and commented, "I worked on the Microsoft's mobile operating system for adaptation to the Nokia handsets when I was in Hyderabad. I was also commissioned by the headquarters to dedicate myself to refine this mobile OS adaptation."

Singh continued, "However, after three years of making a hard push to sell smartphones based on the Widows OS and bearing the Microsoft logo it became apparent that the market share of its mobile phones was less than 1 percent."

Mann Singh reflected on his own career at Microsoft. He said to Ash, "I have been very lucky. The X Box Series gaming is a bright spot for Microsoft as consumers search for ways to stay entertained. My job is secure for the time being."

Singh added, "Ash, the saga of Microsoft's corporate management is far from over. Just wait and see. We can expect more changes to come!"

Like Singh had predicted, the dismal sales volume of the Microsoft smart phones and the stagnant share price triggered a shakeup at the CEO level. Bill Gates scouted for a replacement candidate for Ballmer. After searching for months and failing to find a replacement, Bill Gates decided to anoint an insider Satya Nadella as the new CEO. Nadella was the third CEO in Microsoft's history and the first India-born.

Barely a year and a half into Ash's assignment at the headquarters, Nadella unceremoniously pulled the plug on Microsoft's mobile OS development project. He sold off the assets that were purchased from Nokia for a pittance and Microsoft took a huge tax write-off that year.

That ended the career of Nikola Erwasti who showed a special interest and invited Ash for his U.S. posting. Ash quickly realized that his job is now in jeopardy as he belonged to the group that was working on the now jettisoned handset business.

Ash was astute and he had the foresight to see the changes that were occurring at Microsoft. He did not want to become a pawn in the divestiture of the mobile OS development. He did not want to lose his job and return to India because his work assignment with Microsoft in the U.S. was going to end.

Ash knew the choices he faced under the H1B visa which enabled him to work in the U.S. because of the sponsorship by Microsoft. If he got laid off by the headquarters, he will be forced to return home to his old job with Microsoft in Hyderabad. Or else he should find a job with a new U.S.-based employer who is willing to take over the H1B visa obligations from Microsoft and continue to support him.

He decided to pursue the latter alternative as it conformed to his original strategy. Once Ash is dismissed from Microsoft, he had only sixty days to find a new U.S. employer who would assume his H1B employment obligations.

—

Samir his older brother who was employed with Fidelity Investments in Raleigh, North Carolina has now moved on to a new job based in Austin, Texas. The brothers were close. When Ash narrated the upheaval at Microsoft that took place and his decision to leave Microsoft, Sam advised his brother "Ash, please check whether Fidelity would be interested in hiring you as a software developer. Fidelity is a good employer and is always looking for good software engineers." He provided a referral at Fidelity for Ash to contact.

Like a good brother, Ash followed Sam's advice. Surely enough Ash lined up full-time work at Fidelity in Raleigh to work on a financial software platform that the company was developing. Fidelity was willing to handle the paperwork with USCIS and importantly pick up the obligations from Microsoft associated with his H1B work permit.

Ash was astute to negotiate in addition a long-term deal with Fidelity to have the company sponsor him for his green card in return for accepting their job offer. Fidelity was willing to oblige, but waited to observe Ash's work performance before filing the requested petition with USCIS for his permanent residency.

—

The rocket ride was just beginning. At the age of 29 after entering the U.S. on a H1B visa to work for Microsoft, Ash was essentially lured by Fidelity to design and develop a new financial platform for their investor clients to use. The fact that Fidelity agreed to sponsor him for his green card impressed upon Ash that the financial platform is critical to Fidelity's business and he did not wish to disappoint his new employer.

Fidelity came through. Six months after Ash joined the company and after his first appraisal of job performance, Fidelity sponsored him for his green card.

—

LIFE IN RALEIGH AT FIDELITY was quite different from what Ash was exposed to at Redmond. There were no lavish digs and lofty and expansive park-like settings that he was used to at The Campus. Everything was Spartan at Fidelity. The conference rooms were well-equipped to conduct in-person meetings and video conferences for connecting with remote workers and upper management based in New York City. Open cubicles where the employees including the managers worked were the norm.

Dozens of software programmers and administrators many from India, Philippines and Eastern Europe worked at Fidelity. The caliber of these colleagues was not as good as the engineers Ash worked with at Microsoft in Redmond. However, these differences were inconsequential and did not bother him.

Ash assiduously avoided politics as he believed it was tip-toeing through a minefield and a waste of his time. The junior programmers who recently arrived in the U.S. on temporary permits or were on an intra-company transfer were worried that the H1B visa program may be eliminated by the U.S. government. They were worried that political winds are blowing to shut the doors of immigration for them for making America their adopted home. Ash avoided engaging in such politics.

The fact the Fidelity sponsored him for his green card essentially rendered Ash to become a captive to his employer at least until he received his green card which he projected will be five to eight years in the future. Ash developed immense loyalty to Fidelity for the enormous trust that was placed in him and the extraordinary step it took to petition him for his permanent residency. He regarded this move as paving the way to win a priceless lottery in his life.

The green card, when it is awarded, would be the ticket to Ash's permanent stay in the U.S. It will enable him the unfettered freedom to make other career choices.

Ash's astute career planning and career development by working in America has now placed his life on the path to what he wanted. His thoughts now shifted to his future life, particularly his marriage. He started to dream of the perfect girl to be his perfect wife and enjoy a perfect married life with a family.

—

As Ash was lost in dreaming about such perfect wife, his parents Sunil and Rupa in Hyderabad were busy keeping their eyes peeled for a good match for their second son to wed. Their first son Sam is now married to an India girl that they arranged for him. Sam took his bride back to the U.S. after an elaborate and traditional Hindu wedding in the bride's hometown of Vizag close to Hyderabad. The married couple now has an eleven-month-old boy, their first grandchild.

Sunil and Rupa Sharma called Ash using WhatsApp as they routinely did to speak to their sons in the U.S.

"Ash, you are now 29 and growing past your marriageable age. You are now well placed in a good job in the U.S. and are on track to receive your permanent visa to live in America. Like your older brother it is time for you to get married," they pronounced by taking turns.

Ash protested, "How can I marry a girl that I never saw or had a chance to romance?"

Sunil responded, "Son, romance will come after your wedding, believe me."

Ash knew that his parents went through an arranged marriage. Their marriage seemed like a successful marriage with two gown-up sons. His parents never quarreled, at least in front of them. His older brother, like his father and mother, settled for an arranged marriage and he seems happy with his sister-in-law and now has two toddlers.

Without much further protest Ash responded, "Sure, you can look for a girl for me, but I will be the final arbiter in accepting her as my partner. Mom, let me suggest you find me a professional like an engineer or doctor for me to marry. Look for a slim and attractive girl, please."

With those words, his parents were extremely satisfied. His father replied, "We will do our best, son."

While Ash was building his life in this way contemporaneously and in a parallel universe the life of Sarada Nair was beginning to take shape.

CHAPTER

3

SARADA IS A FIRST-BORN GIRL born to Indian parents who immigrated to the U.S. when they were in their mid-thirties. Sara was born in India and was four years old when the family moved to America.

Both parents were physicians before they arrived in the U.S. Her father Kailash Nair specialized in surgery. Mother Sanita Nair went into the practice of psychiatry after they established themselves as licensed doctors in the U.S.

Ann Arbor, Michigan is where Sara spent her childhood and part of her adult life. This was the only home she remembers as her home. Sara came from a tangled background. Her father and mother were too preoccupied with their professions even before they arrived in the U.S. While in India her paternal grandmother and grandfather took care of her while her parents were busy with their professions. The paternal grandparents had eight children, four boys and four girls who were married and had children of their own. Two of them lived in the same town in India where she was raised, and Sara played with them.

Other than this her father seldom discussed his grandfather or his siblings. After he became a U.S. citizen, Kailash sponsored four of his siblings to immigrate to the U.S. and assisted them financially and morally to establish their lives in their adopted country. However, none of the siblings showed any gratitude to their benevolent brother. Greed of money and sibling rivalry to acquire more material possessions corrupted their lives and they neglected to maintain the unity of his extended family which was the sole legal reason for qualifying for their immigration to America.

Her grandmother in India who Sara was very fond of and attached to died when she was four. Her death had a significant effect on her parentage as she was her de facto mother. She showered Sara with endless love and affection. Mulling over her grandmother's death for years after she came to the U.S. Sara found no relief. She was stricken with anxiety and grief at a tender age.

Sara was an unhappy girl from her childhood years in America. Her mother was too engrossed in her profession to replace the love and affection she received from her paternal grandmother when she lived in India. Her father showed little outward affection and was authoritative. He imposed strict discipline on her after the family settled in Ann Arbor. With his gruff voice she could only recall him saying, "Don't." He loved his profession more than anything else.

Sara began lifelong skepticism of authority. Nevertheless, her father respected her intelligence and resourcefulness. He was proud of her as his only daughter and the first born. Her younger brother was born in Ann Arbor some six years after the family settled there. Her father saw so much of him in her daughter and tried to shape her to follow his footsteps which led him to be a successful surgeon.

Sara hated her parents, particularly her mother. But she loved them, too, particularly, her father.

—

SARA DID NOT LIKE HER given name after she entered high school at the Pioneer High in Ann Arbor. Pioneer is a public school where the majority of the kids were white. About fifteen percent were Asian and the remainder was black and mixed races. She wanted to conform to the fellow schoolmates and wanted to be like one of them.

She had a low self-esteem. She did not want her name to be different and foreign sounding. Sara started to call herself as Diana the Roman goddess of the hunt. In high school she started introducing herself as Diana to her new friends and this became more than a mythical nickname.

Little did she know that the Greek goddess Diana was unpredictable and vengeful? She was a many-sided goddess, embodying various characteristics, from protector to huntress.

She loved the wooden Matryoshka or nesting doll her father brought from an international surgeon's conference he attended in Moscow when she was ten. The figure sat on her dresser, a smiling peasant in a bright and colorful design. She would separate the top from the bottom and nested inside was a smaller doll. And inside that doll was yet another smaller doll, a smaller figure. And inside that doll was a third, more petite peasant still. Altogether there were four dolls nested inside the Matryoshka, the tiniest was one only one that wasn't hollow.

Sara called the tiniest doll as Diana the name that she bestowed upon herself. She arbitrarily attributed different personalities and assigned different Roman and Greek goddesses to the other hollow nested dolls: Vesta, Minerva and Artemis.

Diana was far from slender for her age in the high school. She did not go to the gym or play any sports to burn off her caloric intake. She generally was not outgoing but had a couple of close girlfriends and she did what girls at her age did. She enjoyed the solitude of painting and reading romantic novels which enabled her to relax and occupied her time.

—

At her father's insistence and to prepare her to follow his profession Sara enrolled in advanced placement courses at Pioneer High in biology, chemistry and mathematics. She also took Latin as a second language as her father convinced her that Latin words and phrases would eventually come handy in her medical career.

The University of Michigan in Ann Arbor did not have a pre-medical undergraduate major curriculum. She enrolled in this local college as his father insisted on her to stay at home while she attended college. The university, however, offered opportunities to major in related fields of study which prepared her for medical school admission and helped to plan for a medical school enrollment.

Life at UM was uneventful for Sara. She did not date per the strict requirement of her father. He did not want his daughter to be exposed to young men and the ideas they may sow in her and distract her from the career goal he set for her. He wanted Sara to not lose focus on getting admission to a medical school and become a doctor.

Sara's had little interest in medical study except she sometimes wondered whether she was traumatized in her childhood due to parental neglect. She was wise enough to realize that her childhood and teen years were neglected by her parents. She was never given freedom to do things she wanted to do like traveling and dating boys. She craved for love and affection. She remembered only the love she experienced from her late grandmother.

Even though Sara's mother has been a psychiatrist, she never thought her daughter was suffering from psychological trauma because of parental neglect.

Sara's modicum of interest in going to medical school more than anything else is to find out and understand the reason for the trauma that she may have suffered.

Sara's course grades in the high school and at University of Michigan were mediocre, averaging a B. Her score in the Medical College Admission Test was below the fiftieth percentile. She applied for admission to many medical schools across the U.S. including the University Of Nevada Reno School Of Medicine which is generally one of the easiest schools to get into. But she did not obtain admission. This failure to get into a medical school only worsened her self-esteem. She became angry and frustrated that she was not able to satisfy her father's expectation to pursue medicine.

Kailash Nair anticipated his daughter's inability to obtain admission to a medical school in the United States. Unbeknownst to Sara, he already devised a backup plan.

That plan was to buy a seat for his daughter in his alma mater – the Osmania College of Medicine in Hyderabad. He plunked a million dollars of endowment which was a donation to his alma mater in return for which Osmania gladly enrolled Sara in their med school. That donation covered her daughter's tuition, boarding in the dormitory and lodging for the entire duration of her medical degree course including her internship.

Clutched in his hand of the acceptance letter of his daughter to Osmania, Kailash called his daughter to the family room. When she entered he proclaimed, "Sara, I have good news for you!"

Sara wondered what it was and posed a quizzical look at her father.

"I have good news and bad news," Kailash said. "Do you wish to hear the good news or the bad news first?" he asked.

Sara responded, "The good news, dad."

"You are accepted to a medical school," Kailash uttered in a beaming and excited voice.

"What is the bad news?" Sara asked, fearing the worst.

"Your medical school is in Hyderabad," pronounced the father. He added, "It is the Medical School of Osmania University."

She was confused and alarmed at what she heard from her father. She was confused because her father did not tell her in advance that he was pursuing a seat in a medical school for her. Recognizing that Hyderabad is in India, she was alarmed that she will have to leave home to study in a foreign country halfway around the world.

She immediately asked her dad, "Isn't Osmania University your alma mater?"

Kailash replied, "Yes. That connection helped your admission now." He did not share with her the fact he gave a huge donation to the college as quid pro quo for her med school admission.

Sara's mother Sanita joined in the conversation between the father and daughter and understood what was happening. She was thrilled at the news; which Kailash did not share with her either until now.

She chimed in, "Osmania is a good medical school Sara. You will love studying there. Hyderabad is now a cosmopolitan city with modern conveniences. It now has a brand-new international airport which makes travel to and from the U.S. relatively easy."

Sara remained silent and did not know what to say at the sudden and unexpected development in her life.

He mother continued looking at her daughter, "Who knows, Sara? You may find a wonderful young Indian doctor at Osmania?"

Kailash nodded in agreement at such a prospect.

Her mother's words implied to Sara that she is permitted to date young men, which was a loosening of the grip that her father held on her freedom. Sara was somewhat delighted at this flexibility. However, the thought of leaving home, where all comforts were provided for, and start living by herself in a dormitory in a third world country, albeit the country of her origin, intimidated her.

Within weeks Sara packed up her clothes and the needed transcripts and other travel documents such as her passport and vaccination certificates and took off to Hyderabad bidding adieu to her parents and younger brother.

—

Osmania medical school ranked sixteenth among the medical schools in India which gave Sara some comfort that she is not attending a fly-by-night med school in a remote part of the world. The campus housing was in a quad of mid-rise buildings where all medicos – the medical students as they were called – were housed in individual boarding rooms. Lodging was excellent. Trained Indian cooks prepared delicious meals, some prepared per the request of the medicos' needs and suit their particular tastes at any time of the day or night.

The campus had indoor volleyball courts. Cricket and soccer grounds, tennis courts and an outdoor badminton court were conveniently available for the students. The females played badminton and the guys played volleyball and tennis.

Sara was not much of an athlete and did not participate in extra-curricular sports. If she managed to find an hour or two of extra time she indulged in sleeping which became a rare commodity.

A large auditorium on the main campus housed many activities, social events and occasionally held medical conferences.

Sara quickly realized the medical school was hard. It meant deprivation of sleep and a lot of stress by the demands placed by the curriculum and the managing staff of doctors.

Separation from family and friends she had back home aggravated her. She made a couple of close female friends at Osmania, but none were bosom buddies that she could share her troubles with in an intimate way.

One of such friends is Fatima Begum who hailed from Dhaka in the neighboring country of Bangladesh. Fatima wanted to go to Osmania as the medical schools in her native country were not well equipped to train her as a physician. She came from a Muslim family with a younger sister and brother. She was dedicated to learn medicine at the med school and return to Bangladesh to practice her profession after earning her MBBS degree.

Competition to get ahead was so intense among the medicos that distrust prevailed among them. The senior medicos and the professors took their frustrations on the juniors essentially treating them like goats to be slaughtered.

Physically following the staff physicians and observing them as they made the rounds of the hospital's patient wards hasn't been fun. Some nights staying up until midnight caring for patients became inevitable. Dealing with death on a daily basis became an emotional drain for Sara.

Cramming the thousands of human diseases, the labyrinth of medical terms, many of them in Latin, the too many bones in the human body, and tracking innumerable drugs to learn their association with the diseases they were intended to cure was a formidable challenge.

Addiction to coffee, tea and mouth fresheners became a nocturnal. Sara never took drugs or imbibed alcohol when she was in Ann Arbor. Now she started taking drugs to cure her sleep deprivation. Drinking vodka, gin and scotch, albeit in a diluted form, to socialize with her friends became a habit to temporarily forget her troubles in medical school.

Sara was fascinated by the amazing human body and how every nerve, organ and ligament was connected to the brain. However, her original understanding the connection between the trauma she experienced and its link to the human brain fell on the wayside and she completely forgot about it.

The journey through her medical school for Sara meant making compromises with the luxuries and comfortable and care-free life she was exposed to in Ann Arbor. She decided that this was going to be only a temporary journey in her life and soon she will be able to return to a normal social life. The hardship and failures she faced in med school did not affect her in an irreparable way. She remembered her mother's words years ago before she left home that she might find a handsome young man at Osmania to marry.

—

It was her fourth year in medical school. Her thoughts of trying out a young man to date took hold in her brain. A senior medico, six months senior to her and who was completing his MBBS and poised to start his internship at the medical school caught her eye. He was Raj Kumar.

As a junior medico Sara had opportunities to make rounds of the patient wards with Raj and the staff physicians. She liked Raj's jovial disposition while making the rounds. He had a great deal of medical knowledge and a fine sense of humor which alleviated the demands and stress of the rounds.

Raj was handsome, a bit over six feet two and built with bulging muscles in his arms probably from years of playing tennis. Sara noticed him from a distance playing tennis on the campus courts. His Aryan facial features of a sharp nose and chiseled facial bone structure, light brown complexion and thick dark hair on his head made him look like the Indian Tiger Woods or a Bollywood movie star. She thought that Raj had everything going for him.

Besides making the rounds with Raj her first social encounter with Raj was at a campus party. He was a social butterfly and had many friends. Raj was surrounded by his male medicos who were seeking tips on how to cope with the daily chores of the medical school.

Sara who was at an ear shot from Raj and his ensemble heard him brag, "I really love being an MBBS student! The popular belief that you have to be buried in your books 24/7 while in med school is a pure myth. A decent study of three to four hours a day is enough to develop a good treasure of medical knowledge. Sure, you would have to put in more hours around examination time, but this is normal in any degree course," Raj boasted.

"Did you guys know that the best days of medical school are the day you got in and the day your graduate?" Raj bellowed in laughter.

One of the new medicos asked him, "How is the social life of medical students at Osmania"?

Raj responded, "As for social life, there is no dearth of new social connections that you can make. You get to meet and know a lot of new people, not only medicos, but also nurses and students who are pursuing other disciplines at Osmania.

"Events like this party are a classic way to meet other people. Also, Hyderabad has a number of night clubs which offer opportunities to socialize."

Sara approached Raj. She turned to Raj and injected, "Did you always love being in medical school? How about in your first year as a junior medico?"

"Yes. I have a passion to be a doctor. That passion drove me to handle every challenge, even during the first year of my medical school," replied Raj by making direct eye contact with Sara.

He continued, "Becoming a doctor in my view is a continued process. It is not a single event like taking a physical fitness test and passing it after which you are done."

Raj charismatically looked at her and continued, "Medical students evolve gradually, and becoming better each day with the knowledge and experience they gain by observing and reading. You learn things in bits and pieces and then one day you realize that everything seems to fit in a beautiful mosaic, like the myriads of pieces which make up a complex jigsaw puzzle."

The male crowd slowly dissipated leaving Sara talking alone with Raj now.

Raj tuned to her and asked, "Sara, I know you come from the U.S. What is your future plan after completing the degree program?"

She responded, "Not sure. I have not given much thought to it." Sara almost blurted out the truth and added, "It all depends on what my father wants me to do." She bit her tongue thinking that Raj may misconstrue that she is a daddy's girl.

Raj advised, “Perhaps you should return to the U.S. for practicing medicine which I suppose your dad is planning on?”

Sara did not reply.

Raj continued his train of thought and said, “If you ask me, I suggest do your postgraduate in the U.S. The U.S. offers a better salary has better hospitals and medical equipment compared to India.” He added, “the working hours per week in the U.S. are much less.”

She turned around and asked, “Raj, what are your plans after completing your internship?”

He immediately replied, “I probably will pursue a post graduate course in India.”

“In what specialty, can I ask?” Sara curiously posed.

“Surgery,” was his reply.

“Oh! That’s my father’s specialty! He is an experienced surgeon in Ann Arbor, still working.”

She volunteered without him asking, “My mom specializes in psychiatry.”

The party was near the end and Sara was about to say “bye” to Raj and return to her dorm room.

Before she could say this, Raj interrupted and took the opportunity to ask, “Sara, would you like to join me to go to a movie sometime?” He quickly added “Have you heard of the movie Frozen? It is playing at the Aradhana Cinemas. I read that it is a Disney movie and well made. It is an animation movie if you are into animation. Also, the story is a fantasy.”

Sara immediately responded, “Sounds like a neat idea.” They fixed a time – the coming Saturday, the last viewing staring at 10 PM.

On Saturday Raj arranged Uber to pick them up at the campus quad at 9 PM. As scheduled Sara joined him and before they rode, she changed her mind to see the movie that Raj planned.

She suggested to him, “Raj, how about going to see the movie The Greatest Showman? I like Hugh Jackman, who acted in this movie. In fact, I adore him. It is a musical. We need a musical cure for the stress of medical school. Don’t you think?”

Raj acquiesced, “Sure, why not?”

Sara added, “It is playing at the Prasad IMAX Theater.” Raj directed the Uber driver to take them to Prasad’s theater.

They occupied the very last row of the large theater to watch the show with a bucket of buttered popcorn and two tumblers of Coca Cola. Sara loved the musical immensely while Raj watched her gleeful face glisten when bright light illuminated her face in the dark. She was lip syncing the lyrics as they were sung on the movie screen: “*It’s everything you ever want; it’s everything you ever need; and it’s here right in front of you; this is where you wanna be; this is where you wanna be.*”

Raj gently touched her left hand with his right hand. He pulled her to him and chastely kissed on her left cheek. Sara responded by turning her face and kissing him back on his lips.

Sara watched to see whether any medicos from their university were present close by or watching them in the dark. All of the audience was engrossed in the musical. Having occupied the last row in the theater

Sara was satisfied that there was no one to watch them from behind to see their kissing. It only emboldened her to continue the cycle of kissing that she initiated. Most of the rest of the show they engaged in passionate kissing. Raj's right arm slipped around her upper body. He fondled her heaving right breast and he grasped it using his large right hand. That's when Sara stopped him by pulling away his hand. The romantic kissing came to an abrupt halt after she pulled away his hand.

—

On her own Sara continued occasional dating of Raj. And Raj responded. They made day trips to the reservoir at the Gandipet Lake which had scenic picnic grounds. On another occasion they visited the Golkonda Fort to witness the ancient majesty of the medieval fort in the outskirts of Hyderabad. Hugging, kissing and expression mutual affection was became common among the two especially when they made out-of-town trips and when their fellow medicos were unable to spot them in their romantic affair.

Despite being docile when she was in Ann Arbor Sara developed a sense of dominance when it came to dating Raj. In due course she dared enough to meet him in his dorm room, mostly late at night when most medicos have gone to bed. Her encounters in Raj's dorm became passionate. She admired his impressive abs, sculptured chest, muscular biceps and bulged calves as he undressed. She succumbed to his lead to thrust himself on her. How he managed to maintain that physique while working long and crazy hours as a medico was beyond her.

She lost her virginity to him. Passionate sex with Raj became a way of relieving her tension and stress in her final year as a medico.

—

SARA FREQUENTLY KEPT CONTACT with her family in Ann Arbor through FaceTime. She never communicated to them of her romantic relationship with Raj. She wasn't sure whether it will last especially now that Raj is completing his internship and will seek a postgraduate course. She was unsure whether he will continue at Osmania or move to another medical school. That potential separation kept Sara from even mentioning about Raj to her mother.

Likewise, she kept discussion to a bare minimum about Raj with her close female friends including Fatima at the medical school. Her friends knew about Sara's dalliances at midnight with Raj but did not question her.

—

IT WAS A MOONLIT NIGHT. Warm. Sara could not wait to see Raj as planned at midnight. She pulled a gown over her slinky silk nightie. She knocked on Raj's dorm door which he opened and quickly dragged her in to the room. He wrapped her in a big hug, before gently kissing the back of her neck.

She nestled into him. "Five days is a long time to go without seeing you Raj," she cooed. "I am getting used to you," she continued in a passionate voice. She glided spread-eagle sexually and emotionally on his body.

Those late night encounters thrilled her beyond anything she experienced.

There was no post-coital conversation between them, except Raj would occasionally say, "Sara, you felt so good," after he came. He loved to cup her breasts in a predictable way by putting his long and slender fingers so they fully encircled them leaving her dark brown nipples protruding from his clasped fingers.

The romantic couple occasionally frequented the dorm's cafeteria, which was open 24/7, to have the cook prepare light snacks like *upma, onion pakoras* or vegetable *samosas* and hot chai after their romantic affairs late at night.

—

"You know, girls raised in America are easy. The social life in America allows girls to lose inhibition of their bodies. Kissing of boys is allowed when they reach their puberty. This leads to an evolution of accommodation," were the jovial comments Sara heard as she passed in the quad on the way to her morning clinical session.

She turned her head toward the person who made those comments. It was Raj. He was surrounded by a bunch of fellow medicos eagerly listening to him.

Sara exhaled a deep breath at what Raj just uttered. She instantly knew he was talking about her as she was the only Indian medico on campus who was raised in America. She could not believe what she heard him say. She was appalled and humiliated.

That comment by Raj presumably attributing to Sara took a physical and emotional toll on her. She cried at night, unable to sleep. She lost twenty pounds unable to eat. She shared her thoughts and disappointment about Raj's unfettered bragging with her close friend and confidant Fatima.

Fatima, who is pragmatic and not emotional like Sara, suggested,

"Sara, you should confront Raj and confirm the remarks he made to his friends, because you only overheard what he said. You may have misheard. Confront him to make sure that Raj's remarks were directly attributed to you."

However, Sara was so devastated that she decided to avoid Raj all together.

Sara never confronted Raj about his comments about her to ascertain his true feelings toward her. She concluded that all along he used her. He is now bagging about his affair to his male friends. She was angry and betrayed by the lightness of the way he had spoken to his friends. His words cut into her like a hot knife on soft butter. Raj had irrevocably compromised her faith in him. Her trust in him also evaporated.

That was the end of her short and steamy romance with Raj. Sara made up her mind that she is nobody's pushover, not even Raj's. The romance that Sara initiated with Raj did not reach the stage of marriage well before it fell apart. She lost complete faith in the concept of a love marriage which she read in romantic novels.

—

WITH THAT SUDDEN AND unexpected breakup, she got disillusioned. She had come to the determination she will never again date another man. Never!

Sara was glad that she never mentioned to her parents about Raj when they were dating and romantically involved. By not bringing up her involvement with Raj she avoided building up an expectation of a potential son-in-law to them.

Particularly her father, being a control freak, wanted to decide who her daughter will marry. Both parents wanted Sara to marry an Indian boy from a good family. Family considerations of religion, caste and culture were paramount to her father. Her mother was focused on age, physical appearance and skin pigmentation of the boy. She wanted a male with fair toned skin.

Sara was in her final year of study at Osmania. Her long journey in Hyderabad is coming to a close in a few months. Raj graduated and moved on. Sara did not know where he went and she did not care to find out.

—

THE FINAL YEAR OF HER MBBS program is generally when the medical student will complete a year of internship. Sara was no mood to complete her internship at Osmania. She knew that as soon as she completed her study of courses and the clinical studies needed for her medical degree, she is ready to return to the U.S. to complete her residency there. With Raj gone she decided she will return home without finishing her internship.

Kailas Nair had a different thought about his daughter's future, however. He kept track of Sara's performance at Osmania from the Chancellor to who he donated the large sum of money to buy her admission to the medical school. He knew that Sara's performance in med school has been mediocre, like her undergraduate performance at University of Michigan. He suspected that his daughter may have a tough time passing the examinations in the U.S. to receive certification to complete her residency and establish herself as a licensed U.S. physician.

He and Sani had several discussions about what they should do with their daughter's future life. They knew that Sara is not a beauty queen. She was on the chubby side at least a year or so ago when they last saw her. She hasn't done well in med school and may not be able to establish herself as a successful doctor in the U.S. Given these negative factors, the prospect for her to find a husband in the U.S. seemed somewhat bleak.

Kailash came up with a plan. "Perhaps, we should explore potential suitors for Sara from India through an arranged marriage," he said to his wife. He argued with Sani, "Sara is already living in India. Let us weigh the attractive aspects in our daughter's favor and leverage them to entice a good matrimonial match of a young man residing in India."

Sani immediately responded, "Sara's status as a U. S. citizen may be an attractive incentive for a young Indian man who wishes to come to the U.S. by marrying her. After the wedding, Sara can sponsor him for his U.S. Green card which will enable him to immigrate to America and stay permanently here with Sara."

Kailash replied, "Precisely! That's exactly what I was thinking. The value of the green card is an unbelievably attractive gift of a lifetime for a non-U.S. person!"

"OK. I will make contact with my friends and relatives in India to identify such a prospective groom for Sara. You do the same with yours," Kailash said.

It was Saturday night in Ann Arbor. Kailash calculated the time of day in Hyderabad. It was Sunday morning in Hyderabad. He placed a FaceTime call to his daughter.

Sara picked up the ping noise that her phone made and instantly noticed her father's appearance on the screen. "Hello Dad! How are you guys doing?" she asked.

Kailash replied, "We are fine. Listen, Sara. I think you should complete your internship at Osmania. Your tuition, boarding and lodging has been paid for. Why walk away and return home now? You should take advantage of the clinical training you will receive by completing your internship at Osmania which might help qualify you with the residency program when you return home."

Sara listened quietly. She did not protest as she knew that would be futile as her father is stubborn once he made up his mind.

"I have been deferential to him all my life, why fight now," she whispered to herself.

"There is one more reason for you to stay in Hyderabad," Kailash continued.

"You are not getting any younger Sara. You are now 28. Unless you already found someone to marry on your own there, I think your mother and I would like to work toward an arranged marriage for you. What do you say?" Kailash asked.

Sara remained quiet still. She dashed her romance with Raj over a year ago. She did not want to bring up that past failed episode of dating. She acquiesced in her father's suggestion by not objecting.

Kailash continued "We will find a young man from a good family and who would be a perfect match for you. I promise you will get to meet him and make the decision for yourself. Okay?"

Sara replied, "As you wish, dad."

Kailash continued after a short pause.

"Perhaps you should open yourself up a little to the possibilities around you to find a young man. Is that a reasonable request, Sara?" he said.

Sara replied "Of course, it is."

But Sara knew that there is no one in the medical school she would consider. She conjectured that most guys who are in the senior year at the medical school, now probably know about the bragging utterance of Raj about girls from America. They may avoid her even if she considered them as a possible future mate.

Letting her parents pursue an arranged marriage for her seemed inevitable.

Sara also opted for an arranged matrimony because she believed that parents know best. She trusted her parents' instincts, love and goodwill. She placed weight on their experience and wisdom to find a prospective mate for their one and only daughter. She felt resolute about the notion that if the arrangement does not succeed she can live without her partner, but not without her parents.

Having been emotionally hurt and traumatized by her unexpected breakup with Raj more than a year ago, she still was not mentally prepared to invest in seeking a new partner on her own. Her parents' offer to seek such a person came as a great relief for Sara.

Sara reluctantly signed up for her internship at Osmania.

CHAPTER 4

THE HINDUSTAN TIMES Matrimonial is the newspaper with the widest circulation throughout India. This news media's matchmaking services are unprecedented. Many parents in India who have a marriageable son or daughter use its services to advertise in this newspaper with the expectation of finding a suitable match for their child. Kailash was aware of the excellent success rate of matrimonial advertising in the HT Matrimonial. He decided to use this available and discrete service to find a match for his daughter.

He drafted a groom-wanted advertisement for the newspaper. It read: "USA based high status doctors' family invites alliance for their daughter. Beautiful, fair complexion, 28 yrs., educated in America, now finishing MBBS in India. Family-oriented and loving person. Seeking a handsome and smart professional male with intent to move to USA after wedding. Send particulars with a photograph to HT-Mxyz@google.com."

The response to his ad in the initial weeks of his daily advertisement was minimal. Kailash persisted in his ad campaign, as none of his relatives or his wife's relatives in India were able to identify a suitable match for his daughter in well over two months.

Sunil Sharma in Hyderabad was toying with the idea of placing a bride-wanted ad for his second son Ash now based in Rayleigh. His efforts to find a prospective eligible bride for his Ash through inquiry of friends and family did not yield any promising results. His wife Rupa was on the same track as well and was a step ahead of her husband.

She picked up the HT Matrimonial to check out whether any of brides advertised in the newspaper would interest her for her son. The groom-wanted ad that Kailash placed in the Matrimonial section caught Rupa's eye.

She quickly summoned her husband. "Sunil, see this ad about a beautiful girl who is finishing her MBBS in India. Her parents are also doctors and live in USA. She may be a good selection for Ash. Don't you think?" she asked.

What happened next is that Sunil responded to the email contact at HT Matrimonial. He followed up by shooting off a digitized photo of his son for forwarding to the doctors in USA and furnishing the particulars of Ash and Sunil's contact phone and email information.

Active exchanges of information of the prospective bride and groom followed though email and by phone conversations between the two sets of parents over the next two months. The Sharma's were so delighted to learn that the prospective bride is studying at Osmania in Hyderabad where they live.

Rupa's reaction to this discovery was, "It is fortuitous that the girl is now in Hyderabad. This is a good omen for Ash and for our family," she admitted to her husband.

Likewise, Kailash felt good that he persuaded Sara to study at Osmania. Little did he envision that she may end up with a lad from his former hometown of Hyderabad? Such thoughts were racing in Kailash's head.

He told himself, *"Slow down. Let Sara meet the boy and make a decision on her own before we can go forward with the match."*

Sara looked at the still photo of Ash that her father forwarded. Ash looked handsome. His eyes sparkled with inquisitiveness. The family pedigree of the two sons now living in the U.S. and parents living in Hyderabad was not usual.

The facts conveyed by her father that the Sharma's are wealthy and owners of farmland near Hyderabad which they leased out to several farmers to grow crops and upon which they collected huge lease payments did not enter into her consideration. She was more interested in Ash and wondered whether he physically appealed to her from the small still photo that she looked at several times. She avoided having preconceptions of Ash and wanted to meet him in person with an open mind.

Ash's reaction by looking at Sara's photo did not immediately strike as a perfect girl that he dreamed of to have a perfect marriage. The history of her having been born in India, educated mostly in the U.S. and now finishing her medical study in Hyderabad gave him comfort that she is well exposed to the Indian culture and tradition. If anything,

Ash assumed that she is acclimatized to the Indian way of life with reverence to her parents and exposure to the music and song of the country to which he himself has been exposed almost all of his life.

Within six weeks of the exchange of the photos a formal look-and-see arrangement was scheduled. Kailash and Sanita Nair flew to Hyderabad as did Ash. The formal meeting was arranged by Kailash's at the Westin Hyderabad Mindspace in HITECH City of Hyderabad near where Ash worked when he was an employee of Microsoft (India). Kailash rented a suite with a connecting room for Sara to occupy during their visit.

The meeting between the families was arranged in a secluded and private lobby area well-appointed with soft furniture and adorned with flora and fauna. Soft sitar music was piped in by the hotel's music center to set a soothing mood and tone for their first encounter. Delicious finger food and soft drinks were brought in by two slim and beautiful waitresses and left on a side buffet.

Sara sat directly across from Ash facing him. The parents occupied the shiny and padded leather chairs on opposite sides of a rectangular seating arrangement.

As the two sets of parents exchanged facts about their families, Sara attentively watched Ash. She tried to learn something about his nature based on looks, body language and speaking manner. She played that kind of game before when trying to understand strangers she met in medical school. She scanned him adroitly. He looked handsome for sure and innocent. Ash appeared tall, but no giant, solidly built, but not muscular. He had a warm smile and broad shoulders. He was wearing an expensive-logo, half-sleeved polo shirt neatly ticked into creased trousers belted around his narrow waist.

Ash could feel her evaluating, calculating, and appraising him. After staring at him for a long time Ash sensed that she seemed to make some kind of internal decision.

Ash silently looked at Sara and tied to engage in small talk such as when would she complete her internship, what are her future plans and what are her interests in life. She responded in a soft tone to his queries, smiling whenever she could by displaying her pearly white teeth.

Ash sensed that she is physically attractive and wondered if he married her whether there would a worldwide romance between them like he read in story books. The biodata of age and physical appearance of Sara met his initial test. As Ash gazed more at her, he felt that he is judging a book by its cover. He had no clue as to the details of its content. Is it a romantic story or a horror story? He wished he had some time to date and find out more of her inner feelings and also meet her friends at the med school.

Ash perceived the meeting as inorganic. Both sets of parents placed priority on mutual acceptance of their child in front of them by believing in mutual trust and codependency in each other to bring prosperity and posterity to their families. Falling in love before the wedding was not a priority in their eyes.

Ash recalled the words his father uttered to him over the phone a few weeks earlier, "Son, romance will come after your wedding." Those words stifled any reservation he had about the girl he is now gazing at.

The meeting was cordial, and the conversation was normal and lasted a couple of hours. Both families sensed that no objection was expressed signaling that the families should move forward.

Neither family believed in matching the horoscope of Ash and Sara as they eschewed that part of the traditional matchmaking. Kailash and Sani commented to Sunil and Rupa Sharma that the marriage of their daughter to Ash is indeed a marriage between the two families more than merely the young couple joining together in matrimony.

Ash could not spend time alone with Sara as he booked his return flight to Raleigh the next day. The sole reason for his travel to Hyderabad was to meet Sara and defer whatever comes out of that meeting to another day.

As Ash was bidding adieu to the Nair family, Kailash came up with a proposal after he received a wink from his wife.

He cleared his throat and proposed, "Mr. and Mrs. Sharma, normally as you know the bride's parents take responsibility for the wedding of their daughter and host it in their home turf. In other words, Ann Arbor would have been the proper venue for Sara's wedding. However, since my daughter is now based in Hyderabad how about celebrating her wedding right here?"

Sunil and Rupa Sharma were ecstatic at his proposal. "That is perfect," Sunil joyfully responded. "A wedding in Hyderabad will spare our relatives in India to travel to the U.S. However, wouldn't that inconvenience your side of relatives who I presume mostly reside in the U.S.?" Sunil asked.

Kailas quickly responded, "That is no problem. We have a number of relatives in India who will attend the wedding. Perhaps, we will have a special reception after the wedding in Ann Arbor to satisfy our friends and relatives who are back home."

That essentially sealed the venue of Hyderabad for the wedding of Sara and Ash. Sara was not consulted in advance on her wedding's venue. What remained to be done are setting a date for the wedding and finding a convenient wedding hall in Hyderabad.

The next day Kailash called Sunil to convey the thought of celebrating the wedding of Sara and Ash right at the Westin. Kailash was convinced by the Westin management that the hotel is perfectly suited to host an Indian wedding on their lofty premises which can accommodate six hundred guests in their 24,000 square feet wedding hall.

"Sunil, what do you think of having the wedding at the Westin? Your counsel is important to me," Kailash asked.

Before Sunil could respond, Kailash continued, "I am told that the wedding hall is perfect for conducting a traditional Hindu wedding. The hotel management can arrange a Hindu priest and the hotel's culinary team is equipped to serve classy Indian meals."

Sunil responded without equivocation, "Yes, I have been to a nice wedding before at the Westin. I agree they did a superb job at that wedding. The food was superb."

Seven weeks later a pre-monsoon wedding in late May was scheduled at the Westin Hyderabad. It was the end of summer and was still warm and humid. Kailash spared no expense to have a lavish wedding for his daughter. Starting with printing elaborate and gold-engraved wedding invitations to guests, glittery sarees and *lehengas* for women and stunning and delicately made 24 carat gold jewelry for Sara to wear during the many phases of the wedding ceremony, lavish gifts that his family exchanged with the Sharma's family they seemed to show off their wealth.

The Sharma's were equally extravagant at the wedding. The principal members of their family wore tailor-made *sherwani* or kurta. The women wore glamorous and colorful sarees with hefty gold and diamond encrusted jewelry adorning their necks, forehead, ears, nose, hands, ankles and toes.

More than two hundred guests from the groom's side and nearly a hundred from the bride's side attended the lavish wedding. Sara invited most of her classmates from the medical school including her best friend Fatima Begum and most of the staff physicians. About fifty relatives and friends of the Nair family traveled from the U.S. to participate in the wedding.

The wedding planners at Westin compressed the wedding, which normally takes four days, into a two-day celebration. *Haldi, mehndi and sangeet* took place on the first day. *Baraat* started the next morning. Ash made a grand entrance into the wedding hall by riding a white horse accompanied by a dozen groomsmen identically dressed in cream-colored *sherwan*i attire while loud drums played signaling the groom's arrival. He was received by the identically dressed bridesmaids and the bride's family and led him into the ceremony hall. This was followed by a traditional Hindu wedding ceremony before lunch and a formal reception in the evening.

The wedding hall at the Westin was perfect for conducting a traditional Hindu wedding and exchange of vows as directed by the

Brahmin priest. The altar was decorated with thousands of roses and resembled a stationary float at the Rose Bowl Parade.

The reception at the Westin was a big blowout. Alcohol, especially drinks of whiskey, vodka, gin, wine and beer flew off the many bar stations that were set up for the guests. Merry music played throughout the evening before, during and after a lavish meal served at the well-appointed dining tables.

Ash and Sara who were cooped up in the wedding hall participating in the various wedding rituals and greeting and receiving wishes from the many friends and relatives were looking for a break during the reception.

As the guests danced to the beats of the Bollywood music like the *bhangra*, the cool breeze and the impending monsoon climate of the hotel's outdoor terrace and lawn during the reception was a welcome reprieve for them. They quietly slipped away from the terrace to their honeymoon suite to get ready for their scheduled honeymoon the next morning.

Kailash made arrangements for the wedding couple to spend their honeymoon in Kashmir. He booked them in the first-class cabin on the flights from Hyderabad to Srinagar. He prearranged a seven-night honeymoon package in the Kashmir Valley with a dedicated chauffer to be at their beck and call 24/7.

—

SARA AND ASH HAVE NEVER been to this part of northern India before and they were so delighted that Kailash arranged a perfect destination for them to get to know each other after a lovely wedding and fall in love.

The serene Himalayan range and lush mountain meadows of pine and fir offered them an abundance of beauty of nature. The couple got to know each other and romance started to kindle in that perfect setting.

Srinagar sat on the banks of the Jhelum River where they spent the first three nights in a private and luxurious houseboat. The setting from their floating abode offered stunning views of nature. All comforts and specially prepared Kashmiri food and drinks were catered in abundance without leaving the boat.

They avoided the many mosques and temples. Instead, they focused on visiting romantic places. Shalimar Bagh was a key spot where they took a romantic walk in the Mughal Garden that the Mughal Emperor Jahangir and his wife of Nur Jahan experienced in 1619. The full moon as they glided on a *Shikhara* Ride encapsulated their romantic feelings toward each other.

The Pahalgam hill station where they stayed for three nights offered the most marvelous views of garden meadows and lush greenery where the distant breath-taking snow-capped mountains provided a mesmerizing landscape. Ash and Sara had their best time as new lovers with the days and nights reserved for them for love making without a scintilla of distraction from anyone.

Sara observed Ash as they romanced. She adored his slender body, impeccably engineered nose and cheek bones and full lips. Most of all she loved his gentleness in making love to her.

Ash continued to think of what his dad told him, "Son, romance will come after your wedding, believe me!"

"How true his simple words were," Ash told himself. He believed

that, "*with more emotional investment in their marriage by both, they would be happy.*"

On the last day of their honeymoon, the couple returned to the houseboat in Srinagar which they loved so much. They settled into the boat and were enjoying the serenity of the lake. Suddenly a romantic thought popped in Sara's head. She summoned the caretaker of the boat and asked to fetch a bottle fitted with a snug cork.

She scribed on the lodge's stationery in pen the words, "Ash and Sara are now married. Our destiny is linked forever." She affixed the names Sara (Ann Arbor, Michigan, USA) and Ash (Raleigh, North Carolina, USA) at the end of her message. She rolled up the paper, inserted it into the bottle and tightly sealed it with the cork.

She gently dropped the bottle and the message in it in the flowing stream. The bottled bobbed up and down and sailed downstream as Ash and Sara watched it until it disappeared from their sight.

She asked the caretaker, "Where does this river end? Do you know?"

He replied "I am not sure Madam, but I think the Jhelum merges with the Indus River in eastern Pakistan. I am not sure where the Indus River ends."

He volunteered the source of this river are the Himalaya Mountains, which Sara already surmised as such.

Sara watched Ash as they romanced in the houseboat. She wondered whether she would be happy with Ash and is prepared to spend the rest of her life with him.

She could not help comparing Ash with Raj. Ash is not tall. He is less than six feet. He is not highly muscular like Raj was. Ash never frequented the gym or played any sports that he told her about. Sara concluded that Ash is more cerebral than physical. She felt him adequate and their short honeymoon provided a sexual rebound from her now year old relationship with Raj.

As dusk settled in the houseboat for more love making, it was rudely interrupted by gunshots that shattered the stillness of the valley.

The manager of the houseboat rushed on to the boat and frantically announced, "Hello Mr. & Mrs. Sharma, sorry to interlude. The gunshots you heard came from the Pakistani soldiers."

He added, "The soldiers from time to time engage in harassing tourists and the locals on the Indian side of the Kashmir Valley. I am sure the shooting will stop in due course. Our soldiers will return the fire. If the shooting persists, you are better off moving to a secure place which I can arrange for you."

Their flight back to Hyderabad was scheduled for the following morning which was more than twelve hours away.

Without waiting for the gun fight between the Pakistani and Indian soldiers to subside the honeymoon couple hurriedly packed up their belongings and fled to the safety and security of the airport. They wanted to dash out of Kashmir. They checked into the First-Class lounge at the airport as they awaited their flight the following morning.

This was how their honeymoon in the Kashmir Valley ended exciting as it was in so many ways, getting acquainted with a stranger, romancing the stranger and facing the threat of potential terrorism.

Despite the wonderful honeymoon in Kashmir, entering into a genuine romantic relationship with Ash hadn't been easy for Sara. But there was something about Ash's calm and gentleness and intelligence that worked to lower her inhibition and allowed to believe in him.

When Ash whispered in Sara's ears, "You are attractive. I am so glad to have married you," those words enabled her to drop her inhibition.

Ash admired her full figure and well-rounded breasts. He found her sexy and intimated his desire for her. For Sara the marriage started out feeling like magic. She felt satisfied with Ash as her marriage partner.

—

It was already three weeks since Ash was away from his work at Fidelity. His time-off was ending in less than a week. After returning from their honeymoon, as expected the newlyweds stayed with Ash's parents even though Sara had her dorm room at Osmania still reserved for her. This also provided an opportunity for the parents-in-law to get more acquainted with their new daughter-in-law.

Sara wanted to know more about the Sharma family and their ancestry more than her husband who probably already knew about their ancestry. She was inquisitive as to how they came into the possession of the farmlands they owned. She peppered them with detailed questions of the number of acres of land they owned, how many leases they signed with small farmers, and the annual income from those leases the family was deriving.

The fact that the farmland was fetching nearly a quarter of a million dollars from the leases Sara was thrilled to find out. Her father-in-law told that the land has been in the Sharma family for several generations. Its value appreciated over the years. When Ash told her that land was worth tens of millions of dollars, her eyes lit up and brought home the belief that her husband together with his older brother are in line for a monumental inheritance. It registered in her mind that perhaps the Sharma family is richer than her parents who themselves are well-to-do and regarded as the top one percenters in America in terms of their wealth.

—

Ash returned to Raleigh and Sara moved back into her dorm room to wind up her internship. After a whirlwind of activity associated with her wedding and honeymoon, going back to the campus and engaging in her medical studies was difficult for her. The sudden loneliness distressed her beyond anything she experienced.

She was desperate to give up completing her internship which was less than four months away and return to U.S. to be close to Ash and her family. She decided to skip her rotations in surgery and psychiatry.

Sara came to the conclusion that the destiny that mattered now is with Ash.

By the end of September after essentially fulfilling her core internship and having earned her MBBS degree Sara moved back home to her parents.

Ash was still living in a small one-bedroom rental unit in Raleigh. The newly married couple thought that it is not comfortable for Sara to move in with Ash right away. Moving back into the luxurious and spacious house of her parents made sense to Sara. The couple agreed to an arrangement that Ash will visit Sara in Ann Arbor every weekend to spend quality and romantic time with his wife.

—

THERE WAS ANOTHER COMPELLING reason for her to go back to Ann Arbor rather than join her husband in Raleigh. As a foreign medical graduate after completing MBBS a lot more work lay ahead to qualify as a licensed physician in the U.S. Ann Arbor and its vicinity offered a more opportunistic place to complete this task surrounded by her physician parents and their many friends in the medical profession.

CHAPTER 5

THE UNITED STATES MEDICAL Licensing Examination (USMLE) is the only path for a foreign medical graduate holding a MBBS degree to get certified and start medical training in the U.S. Sara needed to do postgraduate medicine in the U.S. after completing her MBBS in order to qualify for residency training. The residency generally took three or more years in an accredited teaching hospital depending on the medical specialty. The option she faced was to appear for the USMLE and secure high enough score to qualify for residency.

Confident that her knowledge of medicine was sufficient, she took the USMLE right after returning to Ann Arbor without telling Ash or her parents. However, she failed in that examination. Six months later she took preparatory courses from Kaplan Test Prep geared toward passing the USMLE. The Kaplan courses were online videos of lectures by professional doctors versed in teaching techniques. Sara watched them at a fast pace when she thought she already knew the stuff. She skipped through some videos like pharmacology because she knew that material well. She felt confident she was now well prepared.

However, she failed again to secure the minimum number of points to pass the USMLE.

Sara's successive failures to pass this first hurdle thoroughly discouraged her. She was beginning to get disillusioned. Her parents, especially Kailash, were more disappointed. The million dollars of endowment he paid to Osmania and educate Sara to earn her medical degree from his alma mater went for nothing. He was beginning to think it was a waste. Nevertheless he did not lose faith in his daughter to succeed as a physician in America like he did.

Kailash implored, "Sara, you must continue trying to pass the USMLE. You invested too much of your precious life and energy in your medical study. You are so close to passing this test. Don't give up now. The world as a licensed American doctor is awaiting you on the other side."

Those words of encouragement from her father did not stick in Sara's head. She baldly responded, "I tried hard to pass this stupid examination, dad. Any further effort to be coached to pass this test would be futile."

Kailash suggested, "Why don't you try taking the preparatory course in a live setting. I know Kaplan offers a live course in Barcelona, Spain. Taking a live course with other medical degree holders from other countries in a new setting may help you."

Sara thought about it. She has not been to Barcelona and heard a lot about that vibrant Spanish city. Ash was standing by her side.

She asked him, "Ash, what do you think of this suggestion from my dad. Would you be able to go with me to Barcelona?"

Ash quickly replied, "It is impossible for me go away for more than week or so. My employer will not let me go for any longer period than that. I am at a critical juncture of the software development for Fidelity."

Ash continued, "Sara, I am fully behind your effort. Why don't you go? You will be immersed in your training and my presence there would be a distraction and you may not receive the full benefit of the preparatory course."

Ash remained committed to her continued attempts to pass the examination, while being sympathetic to her two past attempts to succeed. He wanted Sara to make decisions about her career by taking advice from other doctors. He did not have any expertise in the medical profession as to how it worked. So he remained silent while providing her encouragement and moral support.

—

SARA DECIDED TO GIVE IT a try. She enrolled in a six-week long accelerated Kaplan preparatory course and started the journey to Barcelona. Kailash made her flight and living arrangements for her stay in Barcelona.

She flew in and moved into a vacation apartment in Ramblas in the central area of Barcelona. The Kaplan center where the live lectures of the courses she signed up for is only a fifteen-minute walk from her apartment.

The live courses were better than watching the videos that she did in her previous preparation. But the professors, some of who were from U. S. and the others were from Spain, Cuba and Mexico, were generally good except that the non-U.S. doctors had accents which Sara strained to comprehend. She wanted the lecturers to make an impact on the basic fundamentals of medicine which she needed, but that did not happen.

Sara loved the inhabitants and the vibrancy of Barcelona and the wonderful tapas bars and shops she frequented. The plethora of museums, monuments and the unfinished Roman Catholic basilica of La Sagrada Familia inspired her and injected a fresh perspective into her life. She came to the realization that there is hell of lot more to life than being a medical doctor.

More than the preparatory course for which she came to Barcelona, the city and its surroundings in Spain refreshed her life. When she returned to Ann Arbor, Sara felt rejuvenated to take the USMLE.

She hoped that her third attempt would be a charm and she will pass this time.

Sara has a great childhood, loving parents the whole package. She was never beaten or physically abused. She had nothing but love and support, particularly support and encouragement from her father. But that wasn't enough.

She recalled her classmate in her freshman year at University of Michigan once made the off-the-cuff remark "*We all have demons inside us.*" Sara told herself, "*If I don't pass the MLE this time it will reveal to the world what kind of worthless person I really am.*"

She failed the USMLE again. Her self-esteem and self-worth now plummeted.

Sara is now thirty years old. She became completely disillusioned. She was beginning to think that she did not receive a strong foundation of the basics of medicine and clinical aspects at Osmania to succeed in the examination. Essentially, she is being forced to start her medical education all over again in the U.S.

The prospect of taking the USMLE for a fourth time and assuming that she will pass this time may not be the end of her troubles. She will then need to seek and gain admission to a residency program in a teaching hospital and work like a slave for three or more years to complete her post graduate training. Getting selected in to a residency program seemed daunting. After navigating all of these hurdles, she would have to pass even more challenging examinations by the specialty boards before she can hang her shingle as a full-fledged U.S. physician.

Her parents did not seem to continue providing their daughter encouragement to overcome the many hurdles that lay in front of her to become a successful doctor in America.

Ash continued to be very supportive. However, he left decisions about her medical career entirely up to Sara. He repeatedly assured her that whatever course she chooses to pursue including giving up her father's dream to enable her as a successful doctor is perfectly okay with him.

He told her, "I want you to be happy with your career decision. I want you to be just happy, Sara. Earning money is not that important in our lives. Happiness is."

—

SARA THOUGHT LONG AND hard at the obstacles in her career path she faced. Given her dismal record to pass the licensing exam, she decided to take an alternative and easy path. Totally give up being a licensed doctor. Settle for a position as a medical technologist.

She opted to get accreditation as a radiological technologist at her alma mater of University of Michigan. This career paid a substantially lower salary than what she could have earned as a doctor for which she was trained for, albeit in part. However, as a technologist the stress of being a doctor is dramatically lessened. She concluded she can have a normal workday with the weekends off to spend with Ash and the rest of her family and friends.

With this decision made Sara and Ash settled into something resembling normalcy. She persuaded Ash to move to Ann Arbor and work remotely from home. They moved into a rental unit in the outskirts of Ann Arbor.

Ash's remote work at Fidelity was non-stop. The firm promoted him to a Senior Architect of the financial platform he was hired to design nearly five years ago and rewarded him with bonuses and salary increases. Every other week Ash traveled to Raleigh to take care of his work at Fidelity.

Sara lost track of Ash's financial affairs which used to be a shared responsibility in the past. She felt their financial affairs were becoming increasingly one-sided. She felt that Ash was keeping her in the dark.

The thought that Ash may continue to rapidly advance in his career more than she would depressed Sara even more. She was supposed to be the practicing doctor and earn tons of money. Instead, she is stuck in a measly job as a technician. She guessed she is earning less than a third of what Ash is. The thought that her earning potential has been truncated scared her. She never felt more alone and disillusioned.

She lay in bed next to Ash after making love which has become a routine although not as exciting as it was during their honeymoon in Kashmir. She lay there all night staring at the ceiling thinking about how her career was turned upside down.

She thought she has been purposeful so far in life, but that purpose is now being questioned by her failure as a doctor. Her eyes, usually bright and focused were dull and withdrawn. Dark thoughts bounced around her head.

Ash hasn't been a workaholic after he moved to Ann Arbor. He wanted to have a homely life with a balance of romance to please his wife and good job performance to please his boss at work. He loved being a software architect. His boss's continued reliance and encouragement only enhanced the importance of deriving satisfaction from his work.

Sara probably needed psychotherapy to clear the dark thoughts in her. Her mother with her decades of experience as a practicing psychiatrist should have noticed her daughter's cognitive behavior and should have urged her for counseling. But she missed noticing those changes in her and did not provide the guidance she needed.

Sara started taking pills to control her mood. It worked for a while by chemically rebalancing her mood. But she got physically sick with the medication in other ways. She then discontinued the pills.

She somehow felt less securely moored to her husband and family.

—

Ash loved playing chess. Learning from his father when he was young and the silent exchange of glances after a move has been made established his quiet communication with his opponent. Chess playing was a positive factor in his life. He developed the ability to visualize, predict and execute the strategy he believed will fit against his opponent. His ability to maintain a dynamic open mind since the opponent had a plan to beat him instilled flexibility in him.

Chess taught Ash even more. The need to defend the King in danger by moving chess pieces with a purpose and to guard against a sneak attack thrilled him.

Playing the actual chess game with a live opponent rather than watching videos or reading books on chess was the best for Ash to improve his game. He didn't join a chess club because it required a certain amount of commitment of time which he was unable to make because of he was essentially on call at any time of the day or night to meet his job requirements.

Fortuitously Ash discovered that his father-in-law Kailash is a chess player. Kailash played chess when he was young. He gave up the game after he became a licensed surgeon simply because he did not find an opponent to play with. Instead, he took to golfing as most of his colleagues did. He spent whatever free time he had by playing golf.

It was winter in Ann Arbor. Kailash was looking for intellectual excitement. When Ash mentioned to him that he plays chess he was exhilarated. They both quickly settled into playing chess. They both thought that they met a match in their opponent in playing the chess game.

Playing chess was so entertaining and stimulating to Ash he made it a habit to drive to his father-in-law's home and engage in playing this game as often as their mutual time permitted. Soon he became addicted to playing chess with Kailash. What started as a game to while away the gray and dreary winter weekends In Michigan slowly transformed into a wagering sport. They bet small amounts of ten dollars a game. The winner received the payment in cash. Ash invariably won. Emboldened, Ash increased the wager to twenty dollars. Over the course of a weekend Ash pocketed close to a couple of grand by playing chess with Kailash.

More than winning the chess matches Ash developed a strong bond with his father-in-law like he did with his father when the two played chess back in Hyderabad.

With months of frequent visits to his in-laws to primarily play chess with Kailash, Ash noticed that no genuine love, affection and respect flowed freely among the members of the Nair's core family.

Sara occasionally joined Ash when he played with Kailash to spend time with her parents. She tried chess with her father when she was ten but never enjoyed it. She felt it was boring and complicated.

With the intensity of Ash playing regularly with her father Sara felt she is turning into a chess widow.

She turned to her mother and complained, "I am a depressed chess widow, Mom. And my husband isn't even dead yet! I am just a pawn, not even the Queen."

CHAPTER

6

SARA VIEWED THAT HER marriage was beginning to get stale. It was no longer generating the feeling of magic it did when they first got married. From time to time they went away on short vacations to resorts in the Big Island in Hawaii, Cancun in Mexico and the Polynesian islands of Bora Bora. The vacations rejuvenated their love and sex life, but they appeared only short-lived and fleeting.

Their life in Ann Arbor became somewhat monotonous. A routine life with both couple working all day, Ash on call 24/7 on weekdays and some weekends and visits with his father-in-law to play chess became a steady trek.

Sara impulsively devised a plan to break this monotony. The plan had a multiple purpose. Break the weekend visits to her dad by Ash to play chess; and have Ash invest more in their relationship and enrich their marriage.

Her most important reason was to find out her husband's financial assets which she he neglected to share with her. She decided to purchase a house which was far away from where her parents lived at the extreme outskirts of Ann Arbor.

She convinced Ash that they need to move away from their modest rental property and own a home to build financial equity. She dangled the prospect of having children and raising a family which Ash liked very much to hear. He did not interfere with her plans.

He said, "Sara, do whatever you think is best for our family. I love you and I want you to be happy."

Right away Sara commissioned a real estate agent to find such a house to purchase. She laid out her requirements for the house. It should be a single-family house located on or close to a lake; have sweeping views of trees and water from inside the house; newly constructed with all modern comforts and esthetically pleasing. She left out the price range of the house. She was open to check out all listed properties which met her lofty requirements.

It was early fall, and the leaves were beginning to display their brilliant colors of the season. Sara dragged Ash to look at dozens of new and old houses over several weekends. They discarded many properties that the real estate agent identified and showed them until the agent identified a brand new contemporary English Tudor.

The Tudor house was built over a year ago, but it hasn't been occupied by anyone. The house had more than just a nice view of trees and lake. It was an immersive experience to evoke the sense of walking deep down in an untouched forest of pines all around. It eschewed the traditional front door. Instead, a pathway ran parallel to the house before turning back ninety degrees and heading toward a steel and glass door encased in a green grass wall.

A vaulted ceiling loomed three stories above. The house smelled new. Marble floor reflected the curving staircase that perfectly filled the inside of the Tudor. The space was vast and as hushed as a cathedral. The library behind the staircase was built with walls on two sides consisting of floor-to-ceiling bookcases. The third side was almost entirely windows, offering a view of the garden with green lawn and islands of flower beds. The kitchen and great room glistened in the sunlight that filtered through the large windows that surrounded them. In one corner of the kitchen was an espresso maker.

The four bedrooms with individual attached baths located on the second level with cherry wood flooring and filtered sunlight from sections of the glass tiles on the roof. The cream-colored cabinets and marble flooring in the bathrooms and spacious his and her walk-in closets with built-in cherry wood shelving for clothes rounded up the house into an architectural wonder. Polished and exposed wood beams adored the high ceilings of the bedrooms and carried quietly whirring ceiling fans.

Sara instantly fell in love with the Tudor. With great excitement she asked, "Ash, don't you love this house? I have never seen a house where so much attention to detail was given by the builder. I just adore it."

"I love the house, too. It is gorgeous. However, the price may be out of our reach," Ash responded.

The list price of the house was close to two million dollars. The price did not deter Sara. She wanted to make a purchase offer at just below ten percent of the list price. If her offer was accepted, it meant that the purchase price would approximate $1.8 million.

The realtor who already prequalified the buyers for a mortgage informed that, "At this price, the mortgage company would probably require nearly half-a million dollars as down payment from you Mr. & Mrs. Sharma to qualify for a mortgage."

Sara slept that evening marveling at her new find and thinking about the down payment of cash needed to possess it.

—

It was Sunday morning. Ash woke up first. He prepared two cups of hot chai that he loved to make on weekends. He came to the bed where Sara was still asleep. He gently nudged her to wake up and offered a cup of the tea. She thanked him for being so thoughtful to have prepared the chai. The chai smelled heavenly.

Sara wanted to please Ash that morning with the intention of convincing him to buy the Tudor they saw the previous day.

After small talk and drinking up the tea, she asked him, "Make love to me, Ash."

She never spoke those words to her husband even when they were on their honeymoon or on vacations in romantic places like Bora Bora. Ash took up on her expressed offer. He peeled off his pajamas and crept under the sheets next to Sara where she was already lay nude. He kissed her tender lips, fondled her rounded breasts, and slid down to her crotch.

Sara grabbed Ash by his chin and pulled him up to kiss him passionately. She turned him around to lie on his back facing her.

She mounted him and guided his protruding organ into her. With full control over him, she slithered her lower body so as to have him penetrate and hit the proper spots inside her to maximize her pleasure. She maintained her movements to enhance her pleasure.

As they reached near coitus, she thrust her body in and out with long and gentle strokes. Ash then took over and wrapped his long legs around her plump buttocks and joined her in his strokes in a rhythmic way while crushing his body into her when they simultaneously reached the sexual climax.

Ash was so pleased with Sara's sexual initiative. He never knew that she was capable of giving him such immense pleasure.

—

As THEY LAY IN THE bed after love-making Sara initiated the conversation, "Ash, do you like the house we saw yesterday? I loved it. Can we make an offer to purchase it, my sweetheart please?"

"Sara, I loved the house, too," Ash said in a soft and gentle voice.

He already figured out the finances involved to purchase the house.

He continued, "Sara, I think we are not in a position to afford the house. Not now. It is beyond our means. Perhaps in a few years we could afford it."

Sara quickly responded, "Once we make a decent down payment of close to half a million, we can afford the monthly mortgage payments. Don't you think?"

"That is probably true. But where do we get the half a million from to put down? I do not have such an amount of money saved. Sara, I am sure you do not have much savings either which we can combine to raise the down payment. Do you?" he wondered aloud.

Sara jumped to the chase, "Would your parents be able to lend you part of the down payment? I know they collect monthly payments from the land leased to farmers in India?" she asked.

"Sara, I do not know their finances. I never asked them. However, I do not want to burden them by asking for money. My parents have been very generous to me all my life. They raised me in a comfortable house meeting all of my needs. They paid my tuition for IIT for years. They enabled me to be self-sufficient and taught to live on my own. I do not want to disappoint them by asking for money now," Ash passionately responded.

Ash supplemented his statement with pragmatic advice, "Sara, let us find a more reasonably priced house which our finances can comfortably afford. Let us establish our family with one or more children. We can then look for a larger house like the Tudor to move up to."

He smiled, trying to lighten up the conversation. Sara stared at him without giving much weight to his words. Sara could only see the skepticism in his eyes as he spoke about the Tudor.

Sara was adamant. She said, "Ash, I love the Tudor. We can afford to buy it with some help from your parents. It is now or never!"

Ash glanced at her hands. They were clinched into fists.

Having made these remarks, Ash did not ask Sara whether her parents would be able to help out with the down payment. Sara did not bring it up either.

—

Sara's fixation on extracting money from her parents-in-law was dampened by Ash. The love and romantic feelings she had for Ash seemed to somewhat suddenly dissipate.

Sara was aware of the insane privileges she received in her life. She was raised in a well-to-do family in a large house. Her parents paid the tuition when she attended the University of Michigan. The privilege of getting admission to the med school at Osmania along with the payment of tuition, boarding and lodging fees for her dorm, and free books because of the massive donation her father paid to the university. Her father also paid for her preparatory courses to pass USMLE and her expenses to take the Kaplan course in Barcelona. She was the epitome of American wealth which brought her the privileges in her life.

Even though she could ask her parents to lend them money for the down payment to buy the Tudor, she was reluctant to do it. Instead, she was fixated on getting this payment from her in-laws.

The original matrimonial plan by Sara's father to choose an eligible bachelor living in India for Sara to marry so she could sponsor her newly married husband for the green card did not materialize as Ash was already living in the U.S. He already possessed the H1B work visa and his employer sponsored him for his green card. For Ash it was only a matter of time to receive his permanent residency in America. Ash did not need Sara to sponsor him for his green card. Because of this unforeseen and pre-established immigration status of Ash, Sara lost the crucial opportunity to exert leverage over his green card and control his destiny to continue his living in the U.S.

The combination of greed and control over Ash's life had an explosive effect on Sara. Her greed took the form of a running train with no brakes. She had given no thought as to where the accelerated train will lead the journey that she embarked on. Her desire for more money, wealth and material possessions intensified. She equated her self-worth to having excessive stuff with owning the Tudor as the centerpiece.

She fixated on extracting wealth from Ash and his parents to buy the Tudor. It, however, dealt a blow to the love and affection that Ash offered to her.

She devised a plan to directly confront her parents-in-law for the down payment to purchase the Tudor.

She asked Ash, "Have your parents been to U.S.?"

"No, not yet," replied Ash.

"So why don't we invite them to visit with us for the Thanksgiving Holidays?" Sara cooed.

"That is an excellent idea. They can visit us first and then see Samir and his family in Austin," he remarked. "The problem is that it is going to be cold in Ann Arbor. They are not used to the cold weather, especially if it snows at Thanksgiving. I am sure they would love visiting Austin where it is warm and spend time with their other son and grandchildren," Ash added.

"Our apartment is too small. Perhaps they can stay with my parents? They would be more comfortable staying there. Let me check with mom to see whether she can host them," Sara suggested.

Sara's mom was only too receptive to host the guests from Hyderabad. The last time Sara's parents saw Ash' parents was at the wedding nearly four years ago. She wanted to see them and enhance the relationship between the Nair and Sharma families.

—

Sunil and Rupa Sharma, as is customary when visiting close relatives after a long time, brought with them wonderful household gifts of Indian ornaments and delicious Indian sweets for their hosts. For their daughter-in-law they brought an artistically made 24 carat gold peacock choker necklace studded with large white natural diamonds, *navrathan* stones and Japanese south sea pearls together with a perfect pair of matching ear rings. They gifted Ash with a blue and white marble chess board adorned with ivory chess pieces.

The Thanksgiving dinner was planned to be a cozy event. The invitees were limited to the immediate families: Sara's family of four including her younger brother, who is now a freshman at Florida State University, as well as Ash and his visiting parents. Sanita Nair prepared a fusion-style meal as she suspected the visiting guests may not relish the traditional Thanksgiving turkey dinner. She made a tandoori-style chicken bedded on mutton biriyani as the main course accompanied by eggplant tikka, sweet potatoes cooked in tamarind sauce, sliced green beans roasted with diced mushrooms and laced with fresh grated coconut, cucumber raita and hot mango pickles.

Sara adorned the artistically designed diamond necklace that her parents-in-law gifted around her neck. The choker looked beautiful around her neck. She had many photos taken of her presumably for showing off her necklace to her friends.

Sara's emotions were in flux. She felt happy wearing the diamond necklace but got bored at the dinner. She went through mood swings from being happy to being grumpy. Nevertheless, she had an agenda. She came determined to confront her parents-in-law. She wanted them to contribute to the down payment of half a million dollars for the Tudor she wanted to purchase. She felt purposeful and did not panic. She decided to take charge of her goal to acquire the Tudor regardless of the consequences of her potential confrontation with her father-in-law.

The conversation at the dinner table was congenial and pleasant with the parents exchanging the simple and daily stories of life they face in their respective countries. Sara did not pay any attention to their conversation. She was obsessive to confront her father-in-law for the down payment for the Tudor. She could wait no longer.

Sara rudely interrupted the lively conversation and turned toward her father-in-law and abruptly asked, "What do you do with the thousands of dollars you collect from Indian farmers? Do you invest it in anything?"

Sunil Sharma was a bit taken aback by her socially inappropriate question. He swallowed the food in his mouth and politely replied, "My dear Sara, we are saving some of it for our retirement."

He paused and added, "We are actually investing to have houses built in Hyderabad."

Ash interjected, "Dad, you already have a beautiful house in which you live. Why are you building new houses? Are they for renting out to others?"

Sunil replied, "No Ash, we are having them built for you and Samir. Perhaps a house in India would motivate you and Samir to visit us in Hyderabad more frequently. Or perhaps to return to India permanently and live in your own house there."

Sunil continued as the people at the dinner table were attentively listening to him.

"The Indian economy is growing by leaps and bounds. We are #3 in the world in terms of gross domestic product by purchasing power parity. Many Indians who now live abroad are returning home for various reasons. To start new enterprises, build new careers and reestablish themselves in the country where the customs, traditions and business habits they have been exposed to before they left home. The pace of life in India is more accommodating to have a balance between work and personal life with family and friends," was Sunil's speech of facts.

Sara's mother was embarrassed by her daughter's question. She asked Sara to help clear some dishes from the dinner table. Sara ignored her mother. Her mother insisted, "Sara, I need you in the kitchen, please."

Sara said with a sigh, "Fine."

When they were alone together in the kitchen Sanita gently told her, "Sara, you asked an inappropriate question. It was socially inappropriate, I am afraid. Don't embarrass us with such questions again, please."

Sara remained silent, but did not feel remorseful for interrupting the conversation and asking her pointed question. However, she did not expect the surprising reply she got from his father-in-law.

That reply quickly deflated her expectation of raising the down payment for the Tudor from his father-in-law. It, in fact, created a new and unexpected anxiety in her.

After Sara and her mother returned to the dinner table, Sunil resumed his monologue. He cleared his throat and wanted to be dramatic. He said looking at Sara, "Many U.S. expats like Ash and you Sara are returning to India. India is rapidly modernizing. State-of the art airports have cropped in many major cities; and travel within the country or overseas is easy now. Posh Western-style restaurants, movie theaters, night clubs and concert halls render the transition of life from America to India relatively less daunting?"

While Ash quietly listened, Sunil continued turning to his son and pleaded, "Ashwin, you and Sara will have a more fulfilling life in Hyderabad. When your mother and I eventually pass on you and Samir can manage our farmland better. Perhaps you both can establish a farming enterprise to enhance the revenue derived by a more efficient use of the land. My only wish is that you keep the farms for future generations to enjoy. This land has been in our family for generations and I would like you to keep it that way for posterity. It has been like the *kamadhenu* - the sacred cow that keeps on giving."

Ash nodded in silence, as did Kailash in agreement who was sitting at the far end of the table.

The possibility that Ash may be motivated to return to Hyderabad to live there suddenly scared Sara. It intensified her anxiety that she may be moving away from her parents and live half way around the world from Ann Arbor in a new, albeit familiar, setting as she was already well acquainted with Hyderabad with nearly half a decade of time she spent while going to the med school there.

—

THE NEXT DAY BROUGHT AN endless rain. Sara brooded in her bedroom.

She felt lonely and abandoned that Ash did not pull all strings to purchase the Tudor. She decided against moving from her modest rental unit.

CHAPTER

7

SARA WAS AT WAR IN her life. She wanted a change which to her meant ending one thing and starting something else. It meant getting her way. It meant getting her husband under her control to meet her demands no matter how unreasonable they are like acquiring a mansion which was beyond their financial means.

As time went by Sara started find Ash to be less exciting.

Ash continued to think that whatever triggered the emotional reaction of Sara toward him was a phase she was going through and can be cured by being sensitive to her needs. He believed their past romantic relationship can be restored. He continued to show love for her by bringing flowers whenever he could, expressing his love for her and meet her emotional needs to the extent Sara could communicate those needs to him. However, she became less communicative.

Ash made sure that neither of them missed Indian concerts and Bollywood-style musical productions whenever they were staged in

Ann Arbor or Detroit because they loved such shows. He humored Sara by driving her to the casino at the MGM Hotel in Detroit and let her play the slot machines. She loved to wager small money on the Wheel of Fortune casino game slots.

Ash depended on Sara to meet his sexual need. When she fulfilled this need Ash found her to be a source of intense pleasure and satisfaction. His love for her grew commensurate with her cooperation to satisfy his need for sexual relationship. When Sara failed to meet his need for sex he faced frustration. Being kindhearted he never showed his frustration to her, however.

Ash knew that Sara enjoys sex as she demonstrated to him by taking the lead when they had sex before. She is fully capable of enjoying the sexual experience. Yet, she is beginning to deprive their mutual sexual pleasure by clamming up.

The mood changes and aloofness did not escape the attention of Sara's mother. Sanita had silently been monitoring her daughter's behavior from a psychological point of view, as a trained psychiatrist, to notice symptoms of such behavior and provide counsel and medication when necessary.

She made a mental note of the pattern of symptoms that Sara has been clinically exhibiting. Lack of focus as a medical doctor to pass the USMLE, forgetfulness, hyper-focus to purchase the Tudor mansion, impulsivity as when she interrupted the polite dinner conversation with her in-laws at Thanksgiving, and the emotional problem of absence of excitement in life and neglect of her physical health. She also noticed a mild strain in her personal relationship with and respect for Ash.

Some of these symptoms made her suspect that perhaps Sara is suffering from a mild case of attention deficient hyperactivity disorder (ADHD). However, she decided to keep her observation of these symptoms in her daughter to herself for the time being.

She feared that a diagnosis by an expert of Sara's behavioral symptoms, if proven to be related to ADHD, may lead to a negative bias in her professional advancement.

She was concerned that if Ash and his parents find out about the ADHD in Sara they may attach stigma to her psychological condition, and it may lead to rejection. She was particularly concerned that Ash may develop prejudice toward his wife and his social and romantic feelings toward her may take the back seat.

Of particular concern to Sanita was that she may be criticized of poor parenting of her daughter. All such imagined and actual repercussions associated with ADHD made Sanita to put a lid on pursuing a diagnosis of her daughter's psychological condition. She hoped and prayed that in time Sara would grow out of it. She felt optimistic that Ash's continued trust, love and affection toward his wife may eventually cure Sara's symptoms of ADHD.

She did not want to discuss with her daughter the possibility that her peculiar behavior may be attributed to ADHD. She was deathly concerned that any mention of this may further impact her daughter's emotional well-being and make her more depressed.

—

Undaunted by the stalemate in his married life Ash continued to emotionally thrive on his work. It gave him a new lease on life. He continued to essentially work from home and exceeded the expectations of his employer time after time. Ten-hour long work sessions interspersed with telephonic and video conferences with subordinates and superiors at Fidelity Investments and quiet coding to implement algorithms that he created have been the norm for Ash. The in-person visits to Raleigh every other week to supervise his subordinates and meet with management was a refreshing change from being cooped up in his apartment in Ann Arbor.

After putting in such a long session one evening at the dinner table Sara asked, "Ash, you have been working for Fidelity for a number of years. I know your employer treats you well and you enjoy your work. How long do you plan to work for Fidelity? What is your long-term plan with your employer?"

Ash casually replied, "Not sure, Sara. I have not given much thought to it. Fidelity sponsored me for my green card years ago. It may take three or four more years to receive the card. It is best to stay put with Fidelity until I receive my green card. Changing employers now may complicate matters and delay the issuance of my green card."

Sara said, "I am sure there is a way to expedite your green card."

Ash responded, "Why do you want me to accelerate my green card? What is the hurry?"

"So you can work for an employer locally. Perhaps, an employer who is better known such as the Ford Automobile Company? You may also earn a higher salary from such an established employer. Don't you think?" Sara questioned.

Ash knew that as a spouse married to a U.S. citizen, he qualified for the marriage based green card. The timeline for getting a marriage based green card is considerably shorter, about a year from the sponsorship date. However, he did not want to accelerate receiving the green card through the marital route as it might upset his employer who he persuaded years ago to sponsor him for it.

Ash replied, "Yes, my green card can be accelerated to ten to twelve months if I pursue the marital green card route."

Sara finally asked, "How does the marital green card process work? I could be wrong, but does it require me as a U.S. citizen and your wife sponsor you for the card?"

Ash replied, "Precisely."

Devilish thoughts started to creep into Sara's head. The thought of personally controlling Ash' green card intrigued her. She has wanted to have control over her husband. The opportunity to sponsor his green card offered the best possibility of doing it.

She bellowed, "Then why don't I file the papers for such sponsorship?"

Ash did not have an answer to her pointed question. Many thoughts about his strategy to earn his green card flashed in his head.

He then opened up to Sara and added, "I have been on the path to obtain my permanent residency for years. That has been my lifelong goal. Your approach will speed up the process to receive my green card. I am OK with it, my dear."

Ash then planted this countervailing thought for Sara to consider.

"In the long run, I do not plan to live in America permanently. Eventually India is the place for us to live and raise our family. Our customs, traditions, and culture are inherently Indian. That is where we belong, don't you agree? Now that my parents are having a house built for us in Hyderabad, we should seriously consider going back there at some time in the near future," he said.

"Let me say this also Sara. You have been trained as a full-fledged Indian doctor. You are already certified to practice medicine in India. If we go back to India, you would be able to practice your profession from the day we land there. If you wish to specialize in a particular field, it may take no more than a year or two to complete it.

"Let me propose this. I think you should specialize in radiology in India. You are already trained as a radiology technician and have the knowledge to read medical images. This experience will come handy to become a specialist in radiology and put you in good stead," Ash added.

Sara listened tight lipped and her fingers bound up as fists. She told herself, "*The fact of I working as a full-fledged doctor in India will be a tremendous boost to my ego and self-esteem. My present job as a technician is crushing my psyche'. However, I will never, ever settle down in India. I will never get away from my parents. America is my home. This is where I will continue to live, come hell or high water!*"

With these thoughts firmed up, she continued on her plan to sponsor her husband for the marriage green card with the ulterior motive of controlling his immigration status to suit her needs, whatever they are.

The next morning Sara called USCIS in Detroit and spoke with an immigration agent about her intent to sponsor her alien husband for the marriage green card.

The officer explained, "You'll need to file the family sponsorship form (Form I-130) to establish your relationship and the green card application (Form I-484) to request a green card for your husband. I will mail you these forms."

Sara confirmed with him that it will take ten to thirteen months for her husband to receive his green card after she filed the application.

Sara filled out the necessary forms and applied to USCIS formally sponsoring Ash for his marriage green card. A month later USCIS in Detroit scheduled an interview which Ash and Sara attended. The interviewing immigration officer assessed the authenticity of their marriage, the couple's relationship history as well as their daily activities and future plans together. The officer was convinced that the marriage between Ash and Sara was not fraudulent and approved the green card application.

Ash did not inform his employer of the accelerated path for the green card that his wife initiated. He presumed that USCIS would automatically cancel the petition filed by Fidelity for his green card once his marriage green card has been approved.

—

Osmania Medical School is a close-knit community of doctors. The School communicated the changes taking place at the Medical School through their annual newsletter which they emailed to their graduates. The latest newsletter that Sara received announced a class reunion planned in the upcoming spring season aboard a cruise ship.

The announcement of the reunion kindled Sara's curiosity. She wanted to find out more about this planned get together. With that in mind she got in touch with her former classmate Fatima who returned after completing the MBBS to her hometown of Dhaka and has been working as a Family Practice physician. Sara has not spoken to Fatima in three or four years. Sara also wanted to share information about their respective families. She called Fatima by using WhatsApp on her phone.

It was a long conversation in which she found out that Fatima has been married to a Bengali merchant. He trades scrap metal imported from the Western countries to have them melted in Bangladesh and converted to new usable metals. The converted material is stamped into manhole covers which he exported to the West. Fatima now has two infant children, and she manages her medical practice while raising her children with an ideal life-work balance.

Fatima asked, "How are you and Ashwin doing? Do you have children?"

Sara replied, "No. We discussed having children, but never got around to it. We are busy with our careers."

The conversation shifted to their classmates in the med school. Fatima filled in on the information that she was aware of. Most of them are now established doctors and settled into family life while practicing medicine.

Fatima asked, "Do you want to know what Raj is doing?" Fatima was well aware of the romantic affair that Sara had with him during the med school and the midnight visits she paid to his dorm room and whey they broke up.

Sara was more than curious. In fact she wanted to know about Raj, whether he is still single or got married like most of her contemporaries, and weather he might attend the class reunion cruise. Now that Fatima brought up the topic of Raj, Sara beamed and said, "Yes. Have you been in contact with him lately? Is he married like most of our classmates are now?"

Fatima responded, "I met him at a medical conference in New Delhi about six months ago. He is a Board-certified surgeon and works at the Apollo Hospital in New Delhi. Apparently, he built himself the reputation as a good surgeon. He was still a bachelor then. Not sure whether that status changed since I last saw him."

Sara asked for Raj's contact information on the pretext she will inquire whether he plans to attend the class reunion cruise.

The fact that Raj is unmarried seemed like good news to Sara. She recalled the steamy romance that they together engaged in while in med school. She could not help comparing it with her present romantic life with Ash. The romance with Raj was passionate and they liked each other's company immensely. The romance with her husband is now dormant.

After Ash threw cold water on Sara's idea to buy the Tudor house, the romance between them got slowly deflated. Adding to this was the thought planted in Ash's head by his father of him returning to Hyderabad to live in the new house that his parents were building for him. Sara felt less securely moored to her husband and his family.

As Sara's focus shifted to Raj and a possible imaginary romance with him rekindled in her heart, she started to develop a love-hate relationship with her husband. She turned into Janus, the Greek God of transition.

In fact, Sara had a love-hate relationship with her mother, too.

CHAPTER

8

IT IS SAID THAT, *"An idle mind is the devil's workshop."* Sara is now finding her job as monotonous and outright boring. It offered no excitement or challenge to look forward to. She chose the technician position as it appeared to be an easy way out of making additional investment of time and effort to pass the American license examination after failing three times. She bemoaned that most of her classmates from the med school are now practicing their profession as medical doctors, while she is not. Her failure to continue a career in the medical profession bothered her beyond any other failure in her life.

The discovery that Raj is still single somehow gave her a ray of hope. She wanted to meet with him after a lapse of more than five years. The class reunion offered an ideal opportunity for it. Sara rechecked with Fatima and ascertained that she, and in particular Raj, plan to attend the reunion. She then accepted the invitation from the organizers of the reunion cruise.

Sara invited her husband to join her at the reunion event.

She mouthed, "Ash a reunion of my classmates from my medical school is planned in two months. The reunion will take place on a cruise ship sailing from India to Maldives. Have you ever been to Maldives?"

Ash replied, "No. I read about the Maldives islands and the wonderful coral reefs around the islands. It is a romantic place where honeymoon couples go."

Sara asked, "Would you like to join me? Many of my classmates are likely to bring their spouses to the event. It would be nice if we can go together." Sara felt obligated to invite Ash and utter the words she did.

Ash thought about her overture for a minute. He is under a critical deadline to finish up a major milestone in the financial software project he has been working on. Taking a week or two of vacation now may jeopardize reaching that milestone.

He politely remarked, "Sara, I am facing a deadline to complete work for Fidelity. I am afraid that I may not be able to take time off, even though it would be nice to spend a few days on the romantic Maldives islands. Besides, as you know I am a pretty reserved guy. I am not the kind of guy who would walk up and introduce myself and make friends. Particularly with doctors, I do not have much common to talk about. The medical lingo is different. I will be a wall flower at the event."

He continued, "Sara, you should go by yourself. It will be a good change of scenery for you from the dreary winter in Ann Arbor to the sunny beaches of the Maldives. You should reacquaint with your former classmates. I am sure you have lots of stories to exchange with them?"

"When you are in India, please be sure to spend a few days with my parents in Hyderabad. They would love to see you again. You may want to check out the house they are building for us. Perhaps you may want to make changes or add final touches to it if it is not too late in its construction," Ash suggested to Sara.

Sara wanted to hear just that from Ash. Certainly, she did not want him to be by her side when she sees Raj.

Sara booked flights which took her to Hyderabad, then to Cochin. For her return she booked flights from Male to Mumbai and then back home.

The three-night cruise from Cochin to Male in Maldives was booked on the Coastal Victoria cruise line. The ship was mid-sized, elegant with a panoramic walkway on the top deck of the ship to be seduced by the surrounding blue sea. This was the first cruise for Sara and she did not know what to expect.

More than a hundred invitees of the graduates of the Osmania medical school and their spouses attended the reunion. Many events we planned throughout the event, starting with a cocktail party on the first night, lunches, dinners and a gala on the last night of the cruise. Plenty of time was set aside for personal exchanges and renewal of friendships of the attending graduates.

The cocktail party offered an ideal settling to mingle over a drink and renew friendships. Bollywood songs from the past decade were beamed into the cocktail lounge.

Sara was delighted to see many of her close friends and meet their spouses. Fatima looked the same in her physical appearance and perhaps more contended with her life. Her husband while dark-skinned and not a handsome devil appeared very polite and congenial. Fatima intimated that he makes tons of money in his business and as a result she is under no pressure to make more money through her medical practice.

Raj appeared a bit aged, but still handsome like Sara remembered five years ago. He was still muscular in his arms and chest which she could see through his flimsy shirt.

Sara had many questions for Raj, but she did not want to jump into asking them until the right moment arrived. Besides there were so many of her former classmates that seem to always congregate around Raj, she could not get a chance to engage in a personal conversation with him. Likewise, Raj wanted to ask her why she shunned him years ago and abruptly ended their friendship.

—

Raj and Sara decided to skip the next day's lunch arranged by the reunion's organizers. Instead, they met at the Il Magnifico Club restaurant on the top deck of the ship. The window table in the restaurant provided an intimate setting. They ordered a' la carte meals of tandoori prawns and Szechuan salmon and grilled asparagus served with basmati rice.

Raj could not wait to ask his question. His fingers drummed on the table. "Tell me something," he said looking straight at Sara who was seated across from him. "Why did you cut off our friendship when we were in med school? You just went silent and avoided me. I deserved to know the reason you abruptly ended our friendship. I have been bothered by your sudden and unilateral action. I still am."

Sara spoke up, "I overheard the comments you made to your friends in the quad. Those comments were about me. They were insulting. They ridiculed me as an individual. I was devastated and cheapened by what I heard you say about me."

Raj was taken aback by her response leveled against him. He composed himself and started to explain, "I remember the conversation I was having that morning with my friends."

He paused and continued his explanation, "Sara, I was not talking about you. I was referring to a blond American girl tourist who my friend met at a disco club the previous night. They hit it off while dancing and drinking heavily. She invited my friend to the hotel room where she was staying. They had endless sex through the night after which the blond gave him a good-bye kiss. She told him that was her last night in India and she is leaving the next day to return to America."

"My friend intrigued by his unexpected experience with the American girl. He never had a romantic relationship with anyone, let alone having sex with girls he met at the disco previously. He was intrigued by the easy sex he had with the blond girl and was narrating his episode and wondered whether American girls are easy to have sex with," Raj explained.

"Sara, my comments were directed to the American blond. I was not talking about you. Why would I? Do you think that I am so insensitive to brag about my then intimate relationship with you?" asked Raj.

Sara listened silently with great intensity. She realized that she made a big mistake.

Raj continued, "You made a huge mistake by cutting off our

relationship. You did not communicate with me your reason for the abrupt ending of our growing romance. I was getting closer to you and hoped that we would have a lasting relationship between us."

"You deprived me of an opportunity to make you aware of my feelings towards you. You gave me the cold shoulder, Sara. One of the reasons I remain single is the devastating effect that abrupt ending had on me," Raj sniped.

Sara was almost in tears at what she had done to Raj nearly half-a-decade ago by summarily cutting him off without giving an explanation for her action.

She composed herself and said, "Raj, I am so sorry at what I have done. I was so hurt by attributing your comments to me instead of another American girl. I was not thinking. My action was self-inflicted as well."

—

THE REMAINDER OF THE reunion activities did not offer an opportunity for Sara and Raj to meet one-on-one. The evening dinner was in a large group-setting at several dinner tables. The two ex-lovers did not get to sit at the same table. Dinner was followed by a show at the elegant Festival Theater where the group watched a live performance by the ship's talented singers and performers.

The highlight of the final night was a toast in the lounge where the host organizer popped the cork on a lovely Dom Perignon and topped the signature drink that the guests carried. Silly and humorous awards were handed out to winners in the categories of graduate who is the longest married; has most children; holds the most unusual job, etc.

Sara won the award for the first category as she got married to Ash when she was still in med school.

After getting off the ship at 7 AM in Maldives, Raj and Sara had the full day at their disposal before their flights departed to Mumbai and then to their respective destinations. They decided to visit the Kuda Bandos Resort Island which is one of the many local destinations for tourists on Maldives.

They took a water taxi to the resort. This excursion reminded Sara of the romantic day trips that they took around Hyderabad when they were dating.

The beach around the resort offered tropical plants and shady trees, turquoise waters of the lagoon and the blue waters of the Indian Ocean. The sea surrounding the island offered an incredible spectacle with stunning shades of blue that merged together where the lagoon met the ocean at the edge of the coral reef.

Raj and Sara sat under a shady tree in comfortable wicker chairs in front of a serving table. Tall glasses of milky Pina Coladas they ordered arrived at the table.

Raj took a sip and remarked "This is fresh coconut. I can taste the white rum, too."

Sara took a couple of swift gulps from her tall glass to quench her thirst. A gentle breeze finally arrived and broke some of the muggy humidity.

"Sara, tell me something," Raj asked. "Are you happy in your life? I mean, are you happy with your marriage? I understand that you do not have any children."

She replied, "As happy as one can be in an arranged marriage. Yes, we talked about raising our family, but never got around to doing it."

Raj leaned back on his cushioned chair. He said, "Once upon a time, we did wicked things, but they were necessary – or so it seemed."

Sara looked at his brown eyes. They were clear and bright as they have always been.

Raj waited for some response from her, a nod or a word, but she was silent and stoic.

That evening at the Velana International Airport in Male' they bid each other good bye.

Before she bid good bye Sara asked, "Do you have any plans to visit the U.S.?"

"There has got to be a compelling reason to visit the U.S.," was his reply.

"I was thinking, may be to attend a medical conference there?" Sara queried.

"No such plans at the present time," was Raj's parting answer.

—

SARA CAME BACK TO ANN Arbor fully refreshed after the reunion. The quality time she spent with Raj rejuvenated her spirits. It added impetus to connive at changing her life with Ash.

Ash asked Sara, "When you were in Hyderabad did you see the house that my parents are building for us?"

"Yes," she replied. "It is a luxurious house. It has all the modern features with many built-in electronically operated fixtures throughout. Your parents are sparing no expense to have it built to meet all Western comforts. I could not suggest adding additional features because the building plans seemed well thought out and the house is nearly complete in its construction." Sara elaborated.

She added, "However, the house is not in an exclusive neighborhood. It is in a congested area with a lot of noise from the street and the surrounding houses."

She might well have added, "She would never live in that house," but she withheld that remark.

The initial physical attraction and the novelty to discover each other's bodies and minds at their honeymoon in Kashmir and subsequently upon their return to the U.S. were unsustainable between Sara and Ash. The flame of passion began to flicker. The vows they took at the wedding ceremony did not mean anything to Sara. Ash placed a high value on their marriage. He wanted to have children and a happy wife in Sara. He believed in the age-old saying, "Happy wife is a happy life!"

As comfortable as their relationship was before they could take the next step of having children, they had to confront a hard reality that hung a weight on their marital relationship.

Sara believed they had a money problem. The money problem arose because of Sara's belief that Ash was unwilling to accommodate her wish to buy the Tudor house that she so badly wanted. His inaction to raise half a million dollars of down payment had a deleterious impact on their marriage.

The money problem arose because of their stubbornness. Sara did not wish to borrow money from her parents. Ash believed on standing on his own feet and did not want to burden his father by asking for money; particularly after he became aware his father made a huge investment to build grand houses in Hyderabad for his two sons. Ash did not believe in buying the Tudor whose price was beyond their means. He had less appetite for possessing material things and place more value on marriage, family and personal relationships. He could not come to grips with Sara's penchant to place so much importance on acquiring the Tudor.

They allowed plenty of space between the two strong-willed spouses to carry out their jobs and neglected to work on their marital issues. However, that pattern of life was about to change.

—

Since Ash was working from home whereas she had to be physically present at work for ten or more hours per day with the time for her commute and the hours she need to devote to her job, she decided that her husband should take the lead to prepare the evening meals, which she handled so far after returning from work.

She complained, "Ash, I am too tired to prepare the meals after putting in a long day at work. Could you chip in your time and relieve me of this burden?"

Ash did not mind the new responsibility. He wanted to please his wife. He utilized his short breaks while working from home for cooking up a meal each working day. He wondered whether there was a secret sauce which he could concoct to rejuvenate their marriage.

What started as a small request to chip in time for cooking meals, it soon mushroomed into a full blown demand on Ash to handle the chores of washing clothes, doing grocery shopping, and maintaining the house. Essentially Sara turned into a prima donna. She relegated Ash with the burden of all household chores on top of meeting the work demands of his employer.

Despite taking on the new responsibility as househusband to please his wife, Ash did not receive any satisfaction of an improvement in their marital life. Sara failed to reciprocate his acts of affection toward Ash. She became scornful toward him. She did not show interest in having sex. She in fact habitually curled up with her back to him when they went to bed. Her attitude toward Ash was heart breaking to him, but he silently tolerated it.

The marriage green card for Ash that Sara sponsored months ago was nearing its process for completion. What remained were the steps of completing an immigration medical examination of Ash and a notarized affidavit of support from Sara assuring the federal government that she will take full responsibility for the financial support of her husband and guarantee that he will not become a public charge.

USCIS schedule Ash's medical examination with a designated civil surgeon in Ann Arbor. Ash passed all of the medical tests that the doctor administered. Ash believed that now it is a matter of just waiting for USCIS to issue the green card to him at which point he will become a permanent resident of the U.S.

—

THE FINANCIAL ARCHITECTURAL plan that Ash has been working on at Fidelity was close to completion. His employer was pleased with the superb job that Ash rendered and invited him to Raleigh for a celebration of the final milestone of the project.

A special dinner was arranged at the Brewery Bhavana. It was attended by Ash's boss and two senior Vice Presidents from his company's headquarters in New York City. While enjoying juicy Black Angus fillet mignon steaks with garlic fries and a variety of home-grown brews, the hosts popped the question.

"Ash, Fidelity is going to open a new software design center in Providence, Rhode Island. It will need an experienced software architect to manage a group of programmers that will be based there. The job requires physical presence at the site to mentor, guide, and manage the coders. We would like you to head that center. It carries a lot of responsibility, but also comes with a good remuneration package. Would you be interested?"

The sudden job offer hit him like a bolt from the blue, albeit in a pleasant way. Ash was expecting a relaxing evening of fun, but then the real reason he was invited to Raleigh dawned on him. He did not know what to say other than asking simple-minded, yet important questions like, "How many employees would I manage, are these employees been already selected and to who I would report?"

The senior VP's answered Ash's queries to his satisfaction.

The visiting bosses then unveiled the remuneration package for the job. It was an attractive combination of a base salary, annual bonus, restricted Fidelity stock units and stock options. The base salary alone was forty percent higher than his present earnings.

He could hardly control his excitement when he heard the details of the salary package. He was ready to accept it on the spot, but bit his tongue.

He told them, "I will need to discuss the job offer with my wife. She is gainfully employed in Ann Arbor and I am not sure whether she would be willing to relocate to Rhode Island. Would it be okay if I get back to you next week?" He received a nod of agreement from them.

Ash did not want to share the news of his promotion and the unbelievable salary package he received from Fidelity by means of a text message or email with his wife. He wanted to share the news with Sara in person. He hoped the news will trigger the beginning of a new romantic chapter in their lives. They can now buy a house in Rhode Island and begin to have kids. He hoped that the change of place may be good for Sara to start a new life with new friends and a new job.

Ash made a mental note to prepare a special dinner for Sara when he got home and relay the news about his promotion at the dinner table. She was more forthcoming when she'd been well fed, particularly with food she enjoyed.

The next afternoon he flew back home and, on the way, picked up a dozen long stemmed red roses and a bottle of chilled Champagne to celebrate with Sara the good news of his promotion. He remembered that Sara is fond of chocolates, dark chocolates with a high percentage of cocoa. He picked up a box of Godiva chocolates. He figured he has a couple of hours before Sara returns from work and he would be able to whip up a nice dinner to enjoy together.

He entered his apartment to find that Sara was already home. "Hi

Sara, how come you are home early?" he inquired as he stepped into the living room.

She replied, "I felt like taking a day off from work. I am getting bored of the monotony of work."

He handed her the roses and whispered, "I love you!" She did not reciprocate, but managed a light smile.

She noticed the bottle of Champaign in his hand. She inquisitively asked, "What is the occasion? Are we celebrating something?"

"You will have to wait until dinner time. Let me prepare dinner first. We are going to open the bottle and celebrate tonight," Ash whispered.

"Oh! I almost forgot! Here is a box of chocolates. They are dark chocolates which you like," Ash added.

Ash went into the kitchen. He thawed out the two large lamb chops that he pulled out of the freezer. Chopped up a couple of large potatoes after peeling off the skin and boiled them in salt water. He tossed a cup of Jasmin rice to cook on another stove. While these were cooking, he sliced up onions into thin long pieces and diced the fresh green coriander leaves. After the potato pieces cooked to a soft texture he turned them into aloo-pea masala by transferring the potatoes to a pan in which onions and fresh green peas were already sautéed with a pinch of turmeric.

He completed the preparation of the vegetarian dish by garnishing it with the chopped coriander leaves. He transformed the pink lamb by cooking on a wrought-iron skillet with a dab of butter on a low flame until it turned its color on both sides to brown and then tossed the sliced onion on top of the meat and sprinkled with coarse sea salt and a mixture of smashed whole cloves, black pepper, cumin and cinnamon to penetrate the meat.

Ash set up the dining table with a fresh white tablecloth, the roses in a vase and two frosted flutes which he filled after popping the Champaign bottle. He served the special dinner he prepared on a pre-warmed bone China plate with the lamb chops and aloo-pea masala on a bed of Jasmine rice.

He invited Sara to the table. The satellite radio was playing soft jazz.

He raised a flute and said, "Here is to the promotion I received at work!"

Sara picked up her flute and clinked it against Ash' flute. She nodded at the news of his promotion and smiled. It was probably the first time Sara smiled in a while.

Ash came around to the dining chair she was sitting in. He bent his body and hugged her to his chest and softly kissed her lips.

After sipping the bubbly, she dispassionately inquired, "What is the promotion you got?"

Ash explained the details of his promotion in great excitement, grinning from cheek to cheek as he elaborated. Sara listened as she imbibed the Champaign and dug into the lamb chop. For her the food Ash prepared was more interesting than the news of the major promotion he just received.

Ash paused and said, "Sara, I am thinking of accepting the job promotion. It is an once-in-a-lifetime opportunity for me. A new place will do a lot of good for you. A new job where I am in-charge of the Design Center will be exciting in my professional life. I worked hard for five years and I am so thankful that Fidelity recognized my skills and capabilities to promote me to this job. I am sure you and I will be happy in Rhode Island. We can buy your dream house there and raise family."

Ash's words of hope and optimism did not sink into Sara's head. They seem to enter her one ear and escape from the other. She did not have the curiosity to find out the details of the salary package that Ash was promised in his new job.

After they finished their dinner, they migrated to the sofa set in the living room with their flutes of Champaign in their hands. Finally, Sara reacted to the news of Ash's promotion.

"Ash, I think you seem to be excited about your promotion. You should accept it. However, I am not prepared to move away from Ann Arbor. I would like be close to my parents who live here."

She shifted uncomfortably in her seat. She paused and continued. Her voice edged with dismissive sarcasm, "I think you should go to Providence and enjoy your job there. I will stay here."

She was not feeling very close to Ash. She felt her life with Ash is somehow over.

Sara's unwillingness to move to Providence baffled Ash. His excitement was suddenly deflated by her last remark.

He sighed heavily, his head sinking into his hands. He looked back at her.

He pleaded, "Please give it a try to move to Providence, Sara. If things don't work out we can reconsider our living arrangements or the continuation of my job there."

Sara explained, "Ash, no. I cannot give up my job here even though it is at times boring. Once I resign, it may be filled by another technician and I may not get it back if I were to return like you said."

Sara's decision not to join Ash in Providence was a blow to him. He was torn between his professional advancement and a happy marriage. He thought through the pros and cons of their mutual separation and what havoc it may cause to their marriage which is already on the ropes.

Ash wanted to enjoy the pleasure of marriage, but with Sara's cold attitude his marriage ended up being a turn off. Ash felt he was dealt a tough hand in his marital life. He wondered how he is going to play it to win over Sara.

On the other hand, the professional advancement was so attractive. It was more than being at the right place at the right time. It was a meritorious reward bestowed on him for his skills and years of hard work and experience. He could not give it up. He was willing to take a risk telling himself "*no risk, no reward.*"

The next day Ash called his superiors at Fidelity and accepted the promotion. His start date in Providence was set for ten days from then.

Sara knew that she cannot manage living alone without Ash's help that she got used to. She was aware that she is disorganized and needs a guardian to handle her daily needs. She decided to move back with her parents rather than live by herself in the rental unit. Ash liked that arrangement. It was a small consolation that in his absence his wife will be well taken care of by his parents-in-law.

Ash moved into an upscale two-bed room apartment complex in Providence to have sufficient space when Sara visits him there. He continued to be hopeful that after a short physical separation between the married couple Sara will see the need to join him. He kept his nose to the grind and continued to win accolades from his new boss at Fidelity.

Sara was more bored. She was looking for excitement on a whim.

Fantasies of life with her former lover Raj became a frequent occurrence. While alone at night in her bed erotic thoughts about Raj began to circulate in her head. She wondered what Raj would be as her husband.

Sara imagined that Raj would be easy to communicate with. They are both are physicians and talk the medical jargon. She already knows Raj's personality and mannerisms having dated and romanticized him years before.

It was easy to imagine her shapely legs wrapped around him and his large hands cupping her breast. She could imagine Raj entering her with her long legs stretched to the point of breaking to accommodate his immense form.

Her breasts and her entire body ached from want.

With recurring erotic thoughts about Raj, she wanted to get in touch with him, but hesitated. In the midst of such thoughts, Raj sent Sara a brief email message. It read, "I plan to attend the Mayo Clinic Interactive Surgery Symposium in Rochester in two weeks. Would you care to meet me there?"

Sara seized upon this opportunity and called Raj. She did not want to create an email trail of their communication for fear Ash may discover it. In the phone conversation she agreed to meet with him although the symposium has nothing to do with her profession. The sole motivation for Sara was to see Raj again and conceivably explore a plan which involved him.

Sara told her parents and Ash that she is going to Rochester for a couple of days to meet with a classmate from Osmania medical school who is attending a conference in that city. Assuming the visitor is Fatima her close female friend, Ash asked, "Why don't you invite her to spend time with you in Ann Arbor either before or after the conference, instead of you going there?"

Sara lied, "My classmate is on a very short visit and does not have time to come to my place."

Sara had a plan that she conceived which drove her meeting with Raj. From the class reunion she was aware that Raj is still interested in her. She wanted to explore the seriousness of his interest in her. If he is not passionately interested in her, then her plan will come to a close. On the other hand, if his interest is in fact passionate, it will drive a larger agenda.

Sara wanted not to get romantically involved with Raj again until she knows more about his interest in her. She wanted to avoid any possible allegation by Ash of her to have committed adultery which might jeopardize her plan.

By design Sara booked a separate room at the Marriott hotel in downtown Rochester where Raj reserved a room for him.

The two met for dinner at the Hyderabad Indian Grill restaurant in Rochester. After exchanging pleasantries and selecting the dishes of chicken *dum* biryani, lamb curry, *nan* bread and cucumber raita, they got into serious talk.

Raj asked, "Why didn't your husband join you? I haven't met him yet. I would have liked to meet him on this visit."

She replied, "He is now working in Providence. We are living separate lives now."

"Oh! For how long have you been separated?" Raj queried.

"Several months," Sara replied and added, "He came home to see me once. I have not been to his place, yet."

"Raj, do you have an interest to work in America?" Sara interrupted the casual conversation they were having about her husband.

"The Mayo Clinic conference leads me to think that you are thinking about a career in America. Am I right?"

Raj let out a bellowing laughter. "No. Like I said in Maldives, there has got to be a compelling reason to be in America. Most doctors have a reason to come here to make a name for them. Others come to make money by working here. Yet, many others come because they were sponsored for immigration by a settled relative and want to be close to that relative. Unfortunately, I do not have such a reason to come to America."

"Would you come if I sponsor you for immigration?" was the direct question that Sara pelted at Raj.

Raj thought for a minute. He immediately concluded that the only way she can sponsor him is if he becomes related to her. That thought intrigued him.

"What do you mean?" he queried with an innocent look on his face.

Sara silently stared at him. She wanted him to figure out the answer to his question since it seemed so obvious. She did no reply other than prophetically remark, "Where there is a will, there is a way."

After a long pause as they finished the delicious lamb curry, Sara wiped her mouth and continued.

"Raj, I made a mistake when I misconstrued the conversation you were having with your friends about American girls at the Osmania quad years ago.

"After you clarified in Maldives that you were talking about a blond American girl in that conversation and not me, I regretted my mistake. I wish I get a do-over."

Raj became philosophical. He said, "We are all captives of our earlier experiences. I don't worry my life away. I live in the present. That has been my philosophy which worked well in my life."

"How true," mouthed Sara.

After dinner, they took a cab to the hotel where they were staying. Sara did not want to be open up her subdued romance and erotic feeling towards Raj that evening. Raj cherished the thought that Sara may open the door for a future romantic relationship with her. However, he did not push his luck for such relationship that night.

They decided to keep in touch as they parted and went to their respective rooms.

—

On her way back from Rochester she mulled over her plan. Her impulsive behavior took over her senses. She made a snap decision. She did not consult with her parents about her decision. She was going to convey her decision to Ash when she got home.

It was late in the evening, past midnight when she returned home. She waited to call Ash the following day.

The next day Sara called Ash on his cell phone. Ash was inquisitive. "Hello, Sara. Are you back home now? How was your trip to Rochester? How is your classmate Fatima?" he asked.

She dismissed his questions by ignoring them. Instead, she coldly blurted, "We should get a divorce."

She waited for Ash to react.

"What?" Ash reacted immediately, followed by, "Why?"

"Ash, our marriage has been dead for months now. I think you know that. We are not excited about each other when we lived together. Now that we are separated, it gave me time to reflect on our marriage. I realized that we don't love each other anymore."

Ash responded, "Sara, that's not true. I love you and adore you. I miss you every day I am away from you. I would like you to come and join me in Providence. We can rekindle our love and rejuvenate our happiness. I am absolutely positive that we can salvage our marriage," he pleaded.

"Ash, I don't think so," was her cold response. She continued, "We don't have the chemistry between us. Chemistry is something that cannot be manufactured, Ash."

She started to get angry. She began to feel self-righteous and somewhat vindictive. She then brought down the hammer, "Divorce is the only solution to our dead marriage."

Ash slammed his fist on the desk so hard that all of the items on the surface jumped. He couldn't help shaking. His heart raced – the pounding vibrated in his ears.

Those words of divorce Ash heard from Sara hit him like an earthquake. Suddenly his world was collapsing. He felt he was precipitously falling into the deep crevice of a canyon with no way to climb back.

Sara continued, "I am not expecting alimony from you. We don't have children which is good for you since you do not have the burden of child support." I will ask my lawyer to seek a no-fault divorce.

With those parting words, she hung up. Sara feared that she had an enemy in Ash, a dangerous one.

Ash was still in shock at her unexpected and unreasonable demand. He had a pit in his stomach when he heard the demand for divorce. His life is changing whether he wanted the change or not.

Ash's face went through a flurry of emotions all night. Shock and resistance gave way to consideration and finally to acquiescence.

He wondered whether there's another man involved in her life to have prompted Sara's sudden and unilateral, arrogant and abrupt decision for a divorce.

CHAPTER

9

SARA TOLD HER PARENTS ABOUT her decision to divorce Ash. She also conveyed to them that she already communicated her decision to her estranged husband.

Sanita could not believe her daughter's unilateral impulsive actions without discussing them with her parents. She was saddened. Sanita believed Ash has been a good husband to her daughter. On many occasions she noticed the love and affection that her son-in-law showed toward her daughter. He was gentleman and wanted his wife to be happy. She was convinced that Ash did not initiate the divorce.

Sanita wondered whether the symptoms of ADHD that she has observed in her daughter in the past have been retriggered.

Did impulsivity caused by mood swings lead to her snap decision to dissolve her five-year old marriage without much consideration to the consequences?

She wished that years ago she forced her daughter for a psychological evaluation and a treatment for her emotional problems. She felt remorseful at her failure as a mother.

Kailash was ambivalent of her daughter's behavior. He was always protective of her. He did not believe in what her daughter told him about the divorce. He first wondered whether Ash has been unfaithful to his daughter particularly now that he has been living alone in Providence.

He suspected that the couple was leading unfulfilled lives. Like Sanita, he had positive feeling for his son-in-law. He was congenial, soft-spoken and never aggressive with his daughter. He enjoyed the time they had together while playing chess and thought the two men bonded well. However, something went wrong to reach the point of her daughter to seek divorce.

Sara was silently pressured to reveal more to her parents. The silent treatment she received from them after hearing of her decision to divorce was intolerable to her.

Finally, she sat them together in their living room sofa and narrated her past romance with Raj when she was in Osmania and how she mistakenly truncated that romance. How she discovered the mistake she made about Raj at the class reunion cruise to Maldives. She finally came clean with the truth of her recent visit to Rochester to meet Raj and ascertain his continued romantic interest in her.

She unpacked the truth that after she divorced Ash, she would like to marry Raj and sponsor him to migrate to the U.S. and live together as a couple.

Sara added these words by looking at her father, "This has been your original plan, dad. To marry me to suitable person based in India.

After marriage have me sponsor him for his marriage green card to immigrate to America. Isn't it?"

Kailash was speechless at the story his daughter narrated. He cleared his throat and answered, "Yes, yes."

What impressed Kailash from his daughter's story is that Raj is a practicing surgeon like him. Raj is also a graduate of Osmania, his alma mater. He told himself that, "*She picked the right man to romance with.*"

With the new course Sara charted for her life, Kailash and Sanita expressed their acquiescence in her decision and offered full support. Sanita believed in her daughter's plan or wanted to believe in it.

Kailash said, "Sara, you are our only daughter. We love you and want you to be happy in your life. It is unfortunate that you did not tell us about Raj when you were dating him. Also, if only you did not have the unfortunate misunderstanding with him and married Raj in the first place the unhappiness of unfulfilled love that you have been going through by settling for the arranged marriage with Ash could have been avoided. I apologize for imposing the arranged marriage on you. I had the best of intentions to lead you down that path, as it worked out well for me and your mother."

Kailash agreed with his daughter that she should accelerate the divorce and start her life with Raj as quickly as possible. He was thinking of her daughter to deliver him a grandchild through a formalized reunion with Raj.

With Sara's consent the next day Kailash lined up a divorce lawyer in Ann Arbor to file for her daughter's divorce in a Michigan state court. Sara and Kailash instructed the lawyer to seek an uncontested divorce as it appeared to be a quick and uncomplicated way to get Ash out Sara's life.

—

Ash was still reeling from the unexpected notice by Sara of the end of his marriage. He composed himself. With anguish and deep sadness Ash let his parents in Hyderabad and brother Samir in Austin know of Sara's decision to end their marriage by seeking divorce. They persuaded Ash to talk with Sara's parents and salvage his marriage.

Ash told them, "There has been a catastrophic failure in our marriage relationship. Even I was unaware of the extent of that failure. I am afraid that Sara's parents will not be able to fix it. Sara made up her mind. She is stubborn. Once she makes up her mind, believe me it is impossible to change it."

Ash's mother pleaded with his son, "Ash, please come home. A change of place at this juncture in your life is good for you. We love to have you back with us."

Samir saw what was laid ahead in his brother's life. He helped him to engage on his behalf a divorce attorney in the Providence area to work with Sara's attorney to end the couple's marriage.

—

While the divorce papers were being drafted Sara received a notification from USCIS. The notice read, "The Affidavit of Support you previously furnished in support of your petition for the marriage green card for Mr. Ashwin Sharma is defective. You are requested to submit a new Affidavit of Support to continue our processing of the filed petition for approval." The notice also warned that "Failure to file an updated and notarized affidavit may jeopardize the issuance of the requested permanent resident visa to Mr. Ashwin Sharma."

The unexpected notice from USCIS suddenly awakened the enormous control Sara had over Ash's green card. Now that the divorce is underway, there is no longer a reason to supply the requested affidavit of support. Without this affidavit, the application for the marriage green card will suffer a natural death and Ash will not receive an opportunity to live permanently in the U.S.

The sinister thought occurred to her that now she is divorcing her husband she should formally withdraw the petition she filed nearly eight months ago for Ash's marriage green card.

Her divorce lawyer, however, advised to hold off such a move. The lawyer said, "I am doing my best to reach a quick settlement on grounds of incompatibility. The divorce process may take a couple of months. I advise you to wait until the divorce papers have been executed by both parties and the marriage is dissolved before taking any action on Ash's green card application."

The enormity of power that Sara possessed over Ash' immigration status started to slowly turn the wheels in her head. She wanted to arrange her new world in accordance with her preference by using the immense power she wielded over him. She wanted to banish her soon-to-be ex-husband from the U.S.

Her anger toward her ex-husband grew so intense that she was prepared to totally destroy his career, his life and his continued ability to live in the U.S. She wanted the U.S. authorities to have him locked up or completely deported and banished from ever reentering the country.

Sara had perverted fantasies of a new husband who would be the prince charming who would save her failures in life as a daughter, a physician and as a motherless wife. She began to have an obsession to have all records, history and everything about Ash expunged so her new husband would find out nothing more about him.

She believed in Nemesis the Greek goddess of retribution. She wanted retribution against Ash even though he had done nothing to deserve it.

—

Ash held a H1B visa while awaiting an adjustment of his status from this temporary visa to his green card. He was under the belief that the petition for his green card filed by Sara will be completed any day now and that he will become a permanent resident of the U.S. He was unaware of the defect in the Affidavit of Support that USCIS notified Sara about.

Ash also relied on the sponsorship that Fidelity made years earlier for an adjustment from the H1B visa to the green card. Ash relied on his employer sponsorship as a back-up measure.

Unfortunately, and unbeknownst to Ash his employer inadvertently failed to file the necessary paperwork with the U.S. governmental agencies. Fidelity was required to have filed an application for Ash's newly created job in Providence by submitting a Labor Conditions Approval with the U.S. Department of Labor. Fidelity dropped the ball by failing to file for the LCA. Fidelity also inadvertently failed to apply to USCIS for an extension of Ash's H1B after it expired.

Ash became aware of these blunders by his employer when he

received a Notice of Appeal from the USCIS informing that his H1B visa expired over a month ago. He kicked himself for taking his eyes off of the H1B visa expiration date which he never did before. Ash's immersion in his new job and the stress of the unexpected demand for divorce by Sara distracted him from his generally laser-like focus on his visa status. It upended his life more than the divorce that Sara whacked him with.

Ash conjectured that Sara might have withdrawn the petition she filed for his marriage green card immediately after her decision to file for divorce. He figured that her petition is antithetical to the marriage green card following her move to divorce him.

Ash was suddenly caught in a tight spot with the immigration authorities. He began to chart a course of action to overcome his visa issues by conferring with Samir and consulting with an immigration attorney his brother hired for him.

In the meanwhile, the divorce documents were finalized and approved by the court in Ann Arbor where the divorce proceedings were initiated. Ash received the documents already executed by Sara for affixing his signature. Ash signed off on his marriage dissolution which ended a sad chapter of a failed marriage in his life.

Ash raced against time. His only authorization to remain in the U.S. is under his H1B visa. However, that visa expired. The law allowed him a grace period of sixty days from his H1B's expiration date. It is now the fiftieth day of that time period, which meant he is compelled to make hard decisions on his immigration situation in ten days.

He faced tough choices. One choice is continue to work in his present job in which case it would pose big problems for his employer and him even if Fidelity willingly corrected its mistake in failing to file the paperwork. The second choice is for Ash to file with USCIS a Notice of Appeal to the expired H1B visa and await the decision for an uncertain period while not being permitted to work. Neither of these choices appealed to him.

The third choice he faced is to voluntarily leave the country; and return to Hyderabad. He can then look for another job opportunity in the U.S. and return on a new H1B work permit. He did not want to burn his bridges with USCIS. This meant Ash should abide by the restrictions on his temporary visa permit and leave the country. He dearly wanted to return to America at a later date after the storm he faced passed.

Ash was tired and exhausted mentally and physically. It was the most stressful period in his life. The trauma of divorce had a searing impact on him. His world is rapidly going downhill. He longed for the good old days when life was simpler, and people behaved better.

The rapid and unexpected and simultaneous transitions in his marital and professional lives gave rise to the nostalgia of going home. His mother's kind words of invitation to return home to Hyderabad offered a source of communal strength in this difficult time.

He decided he needed a change of place, a change of people and a change in pace to think through what he wants to do next and how to restart his life.

He notified Fidelity of his decision to quit his job. He unwound his obligations with his landlord to terminate the lease on his apartment unit. He paid a short visit with Samir and his family in Austin. With a one-way plane ticket he purchased, he set out to temporarily return to Hyderabad before the grace period of his H1B visa expired.

—

Following the divorce Sara would not rest easy. She took the overt step of notifying USCIS that her marriage with Ash ended and she does not plan to furnish the requested Affidavit of Support for the petition of marriage green card to her ex-husband.

She assumed that her ex-husband will continue his job and to live in the U.S. based on his H1B visa. She was unaware his H1B expired and the related consequences he faced. Certainly, she was unaware of Ash's impending departure from the country.

Her idle and vindictive mind continued to conceive other offensive actions against Ash. Like Penelope in Homer's book of Odyssey the supposedly docile wife with marital fidelity Sara weaved her chicanery to outsmart the brightest male in her life.

She lost her moral compass.

She was in the mood for a kind of jiu-jitsu to control his divorced husband in to submission. She wanted her future life with Raj to be protected against any allegations of adultery, even though such allegations were not made by Ash during the divorce proceedings. Sara devised what she thought as a fool-proof plan to permanently get Ash out of her life by having him permanently locked up in jail.

CHAPTER 10

IT WAS 11 O' CLOCK ON a busy Monday morning at the United States Secret Service Headquarters in Washington, D.C. Linda Barr the main receptionist was busy answering the phones. When the phone rang, Linda answered in her usual courteous manner.

"Hello, this is the U.S. Secret Service Headquarters. How can I help direct your call?"

The other voice on the phone responded, "This is Dr. Sara Nair. I am calling from Ann Arbor, Michigan. May I speak with a Secret Service agent please?"

Linda responded, "So I can direct you to the right agent, may I ask you a couple of questions?"

Sara said, "Yes."

Linda asked, "What prompted you to speak with a Secret Service agent? Is it a Freedom of Information Act matter, counterfeit currency, or a threat against an elected official? If you could be specific, I can channel your call to the right agent."

Sara replied, "It is regarding a threat made against the president of the United States."

Linda said, "OK. That is specific enough. Hold on as I find an available agent."

Thirty seconds elapsed. Linda came back on the line to reply the caller.

Linda said, "Hello Doctor. Let me put you through agent Sarkssian. He works in our Protective Intelligence and Threat Assessment department. He will be able to assist you."

Linda made the connection while remaining on the phone line to ensure that she connected the caller with Mr. Sarkissian.

Sarkissian started with, "Hello, I am a special agent. My name is Michael Sarkissian. How may I help you?"

Sara coolly responded, "Hello. I would like to report a threat made against the president of the United States."

The agent interrupted and advised, "You are speaking to me on a secure phone line because of the sensitivity of the matter. This conversation is being recorded. Are you OK with this?"

"Yes," replied Sara.

After gathering the basic information about the caller and the subject who made the alleged threat such as name, address, date of birth, social security number, phone, email, Sarkissian attempted to launch into a series of detailed questions for the caller.

Sara interrupted him and wanted to provide additional information.

She said, "I think it will help if you know more about the threat."

Without waiting for a response, she continued to say, "The subject is my ex-husband. We got divorced a few days ago after more than five years of marriage. We have been separated for many months.

"He lives in Providence, Rhode Island. I live in Ann Arbor, Michigan. He was not in favor of a divorce. When I told him that we should get a divorce, my ex-husband became furious. He then made a threat over the phone that he will kill the president if you go through with the divorce."

"Doctor, have you contacted your local police or the FBI to report the threat?" asked Sarkissian.

"No. I read somewhere that it is the Secret Service's role to protect the president. That is why I am calling you directly," was her response.

"How do you know of the threat that the individual made?" asked Sarkissian.

The special agent appeared to be reading off of a list of questions from a manual.

The caller responded, "Like I said, he pointedly made the threat directly over the phone to me."

"What is the individual's motive to assassinate the president? How did he develop the idea of assassination?" asked Sarkiussian.

She responded, "I do not know. Like I stated the divorce may have triggered the threat of violence. I know he did not want a divorce. He was unhappy with the divorce proceedings. Perhaps the assassination was an acceptable solution in his mind for the unwanted divorce."

The Secret Service special agent asked, "Does he possess a weapon to assassinate the president?"

Sarkissian then added a related question, "Has he received weapon's training?"

She replied, "He did not possess a gun when we lived together. May be that has changed since we were separated and living apart in different states. He lives in Rhode Island, I live in Michigan, you know. I don't know whether he received any training to use guns."

Agent Sarkissian queried, "What is his plan of attack? Did he make any specific communication to you or others regarding his planned attack?"

She responded, "I don't know, but he is fixated on the president. He did not reveal to me a plan of attack, nor did I ask for such a plan."

Sarkissian tried to probe more and asked, "Did he have any grievance or resentment against the president?"

"No, not that he told me about," was Sara's reply.

Sarkissian asked another question, "Does the individual have any symptoms of mental illness which might have played a role into threatening the president?"

"I don't think so. But again I do not know what effect the divorce had on his mental state," was her reply.

She paused and returned with an additional piece of information which she did not relay earlier.

"I just remembered. My ex-husband said that if you go through with the divorce the president will be dead in a week after the divorce," she said.

Sarkissian specifically questioned, "When exactly did you both get divorced?"

Sara quickly replied, "Exactly ten days ago."

Sarkission realized that the threat made by the subject to kill the president in a week after the divorce did not materialize. He wondered whether the subject made an idle threat.

The agent paused for a moment and appraised her, "Doctor, I am asking these detailed questions to make an assessment of the threat. The information you provide would help us make the assessment and take measures to protect the president and prevent harm to him."

Sara voluntarily and hastily added the information about her ex-husband's immigration status.

She said, "I sponsored my ex-husband for a marriage green card so he could permanently live in the U.S. However, after our divorce took effect, I withdrew that sponsorship. I do not know his immigration status now. Perhaps, he is now an illegal alien. He may kill the president and then flee the country."

The agent asked a series of detailed questions and gathered from her information about her ex-husband's employment history, criminal records and history of violence to the extent she was aware of and willing to share such data.

Sarkissian looked at his watch. He was talking to the caller for over ninety minutes. He decided to stop the interview.

He finally said, "Doctor, I would like to stop my questions for now. Thanks for calling the Secret Service. You have done the right thing. The Secret Service takes all reported credible threats of our political leaders very seriously. We will talk again after I make an initial assessment of the credibility of the threat. Thank you very much. Have a good day."

—

SARA DEVELOPED AN EVIL and depraved status of mind to have reported a falsified threat by her former husband against the life of the president. She demonstrated a conscious disregard for his life which has already been shattered by the divorce that she demanded and reached.

—

AFTER HE HUNG UP THE phone the special agent Sarkissian opened a case. The purpose of the case is to identify, analyze and manage the person who posed a threat to the protected official.

Sarkissian had the law on his back to do what he needed to do. The USA Patriot's Act of 2001 provided the tools needed to intercept and obstruct terrorism. The Act provided the FBI, CIA, and NSA to carry out domestic surveillance. Under these powers the government can look at records of an individual's activity held by third parties such as an employer or local law enforcement agency. It can search private property without notice to the owner; it can collect foreign intelligence information; and through spying collect the origin and destination of communications. The Patriot's Act also gave power to detain non-citizens for an indefinite period.

The Secret Service agent started to develop a plan to assess the threat. The Secret Service generally depends on the cooperation, information and assistance from many government agencies. He listed USCIS, NSA, FBI, State and local Police, Education, and Employer as his initial order of inquiry.

Sarkissian realized he needs someone to assist him with the assessment. "*No individual, no matter how good, could be as good as a team*," he told himself.

He lined up another Secret Service agent James Puller. Jim helped him in the past with similar investigations. Jim is a computer nerd and has many friends from his college years at MIT who worked for the National Security Agency. Another former classmate and friend with whom Jim rock climbed occasionally also now worked at NSA. Sarkissian envisioned that his investigation will require NSA's assistance. Jim's access to this secretive Agency through his classmates and friends would be helpful to speed up his investigation.

Thanks to the marvels of the digital age, data that captures the behavior of individuals in their daily life is now stored in one database or another under the Patriot's Act. Retrieval of the data is quick and happens with a few strokes on a computer keyboard. Piecing together the bits of retrieved data into a connected mosaic is the challenge Sarkissian will face.

Sarkissian right away contacted USCIS and requested an up-to-date report on the history of the subject's immigration status.

Within forty-eight hours a comprehensive report arrived in the form of an electronic file. It indicated that Ash's immigration status is in a limbo. His green card application filed by his former wife has been withdrawn and is defunct now. The green card application filed for him by his employer (Fidelity Investments) went into a limbo because of his wife's subsequent application filed for the marriage green card. His H1B visa expired nearly fifty-five days ago. He has only two days of grace period remaining to apply for a renewal of his H1B work permit or file other appeals to the USCIS. If he failed to take one of these measures, the report concluded that his continued stay in the U.S. would be a violation of the U.S. immigration laws.

Per Sarkissian's plan, Jim Puller worked to gather intelligence that was needed from NSA, which is known to selectively monitor phone calls made or received from domestic and foreign terrorists. Jim was tasked to persuade his buddies at NSA to track down the recorded phone chatter involving Ash Sharma's phone that may have occurred over the past six months.

NSA reported that Ash was never in NSA's line of sight for monitoring phone chatter. However, the Agency did not rule out that the subject could be part of a sleeper cell associated with a terrorist group based overseas which may have a devious plan to attack the president or cause destruction to U.S. property.

Armed with these reports, Sarkissian proactively launched an urgent inquiry of Ash's physical whereabouts and his immediate plans. Using the enormous established power that the Secret Service has as part of FBI Joint Terrorism Task Force, the special agent requested the FBI and the local police agencies in Redmond, Raleigh, Ann Arbor and Providence to conduct an urgent and exhaustive investigation of Ash. Sarkissian directed the agencies to investigate the subject's life structure and background including the history of education, criminal activity, marital and other relationships, employment, travel and mental health.

The deep power of the Secret Service Agency netted results in a record time. The FBI and police reports indicated no manifestation of interest about murder or assassination, no evidence that he was thinking about or planning an attack on the president. The reports were benign with no reported history of any crime or violence.

The employment history identified that Ash worked at Microsoft in Redmond and at Fidelity in Raleigh and Providence. The history also reported that he quit his job at Fidelity a few days ago.

The report also alerted that Ash is scheduled to close up his apartment lease and bank account in a day or two.

Sarkissian called Sara on the phone and asked, “Do you know what your ex-husband’s plan might be to carry out the threat he made?”

She had no information about her ex-husband’s plans and was of no help to the agent.

She said, “I have not spoken with him since he communicated the threat. My lawyer has been handling the divorce papers with his lawyer. That’s all.”

The next morning the Secret Service agent decided to check with the manifests of all major airlines to find out whether the subject’s name was listed as a passenger on their international flights - particularly those flights bound for India as the final destination point. This was a tedious and time-consuming process driven by data gathering from dozens of airlines that fly every day from dozens of gateway airports in the U.S. Some flights go directly and others through connecting flights to cities in India.

He waited. At about 5 PM Sarkissian inquiry of the airline manifests netted the surprising result: Ash Sharma is listed as a passenger on a flight scheduled to depart from the Newark International Airport this afternoon. It is United Airlines flight 801 which is a non-stop flight bound for New Delhi. The flight is scheduled to depart at 9:07 PM.

Sarkissian called United Airlines and confirmed that Ash has a reservation on flight 801. He wanted to request the Captain of flight 801to delay the flight's departure until the law enforcement authorities removed a fleer from the plane he will command. However, he was unable to contact the Captain. He decided to reach the Captain later that evening.

Sarkissian looked at his watch. It showed 6 PM. He has only three hours before the flight will leave the U.S.

Sarkissian scrambled to stop the fleeing passenger from leaving the country. He wanted to personally talk with him about the threat. He wasn't sure whether India signed an extradition treaty with the U.S. to have Ash extradited back to the U.S. once he reached India. He didn't want to get caught up in a diplomatic tussle with the Indian government. He needed to act fast and stop the accused from leaving the country.

He contacted the head of New York branch of the FBI as well as the Port Authority Police and scheduled a conference call with them to stop the passenger from taking the identified United Airlines light.

In the conference call Sarkissian identified the subject of his investigation and briefed them of the nature and gravity of the threat.

Sarkissian's message to the law enforcement agencies was clear. It was, "The subject passenger has not committed a crime that I am aware of. I merely want to question him. If the subject boarded the flight, please detain him at the airport. Please make sure that no bodily harm is caused to him in your effort to detain him. Please report to me after you got him off the plane and he is in your custody. I will then fly up to Newark to question him."

The Port Authority Police quickly backed out of getting involved without giving a reason. In effect, the Port Authority Police delegated to the FBI to handle the detention.

The FBI head identified during the conference call that Frank Tilson and Bud Gibson, who are also based in New York, as the agents assigned to handle the detention. Tilson was already present on the call along with his boss and listened to the briefing made by Sarkissian.

Sarkissian directly addressed the FBI agent reemphasizing, "Mr. Tilson, I must interview the subject and get some vital information from him. Please detain him for that purpose. If he did not embark the flight, then we many need a manhunt to find him."

The 3-way conference call ended with that directive from Sarkissian.

—

A FACE-TO-FACE INTERVIEW with Ash was critical to Sarkissian. He wanted to understand Ash's thinking and behavior to have made the violent threat to kill the president.

As the Secret Service agent waited for the subject's detention, Sarkissian looked back at how the potential threat was spotted. The information that Dr. Sara Nair provided in her phone call with him appeared on the surface to be innocuous. The thought occurred to Sarkissian that the informant may have been biased and the reported threat may have been concocted. Perhaps, it stemmed from an unhappy and bitter relationship with her divorced husband. He wondered could this be the case of a divorced wife taking revenge against her former husband by publicly humiliating him.

He set that thought aside. He took the reported threat of violent terrorism, which is what the threat to assassinate the president of the United States is, very seriously as he should. He carried out his mission to assess the threat before reaching a conclusion and take further action to protect the president. He remembered his pledge to the Secret Service Agency to take the bullet to protect the president and his family.

—

It was past 9 PM. Sarkissian's cell phone vibrated. It was Frank Tilson. Sarkissian answered by swiping his phone and listened.

"We have the subject under the FBI custody. Everything went smoothly. The subject did not resist. We are taking him to a secure area of the Newark Airport's TSA facilities. What is your plan to interview him?" asked Tilson.

Sarkissian replied, "Great news! I have been monitoring the schedules of civilian flights from Regan Airport to the New York area. An available flight is on Southwest from here to La Guardia departing at 9:50 pm which will arrive in New York around 11 PM. My colleague Jim Puller and I will take that flight. We are close to the Regan airport now. I will call you as soon we land in New York."

"In the meanwhile, what shall we do with the subject?" asked Tilson.

"Interrogate him as you normally do after an arrest. Isn't it what you are required to do? I need a report from you anyway detailing your detention and the information you gathered from the detainee."

"Will do," Tilson responded before he switched off his cell phone.

CHAPTER 11

ASH'S EJECTION FROM THE delayed United Airlines flight was quick and smooth and professionally handled. After emerging from the jet bridge into throngs of passengers, the disembarkation looked like a gentleman's escort with no reason for anyone to suspect that Ash was under arrest or forcibly being removed from the plane. He was not harassed during the apprehension. Ash fully cooperated and complied with the FBI agent's directions.

He was led down a set of stairs to a room with a low ceiling in the basement inside the TSA facilities of the airport. The room was cold with no semblance of any heat turned on for a while.

Ash was ushered to take a seat in front of a large foldable metal table. The two FBI agents took seats across the table directly in front of him.

The agents identified themselves.

"I am Supervisory Special Agent Frank Tilson with the Federal

Bureau of Investigation," said the man who had been communicating with him on the plane.

Tilson added, "My colleague next to me is Special Agent Bud Gibson." Gibson nodded his head to Ash.

Ash watched cop shows on the TV and wondered whether the federal agents were going to read his Miranda rights. He stared at them. Tilson took the cue. Before he began the custodial interrogation, he read the Miranda magic words, "You have the right to remain silent. Anything you say can and will be used against you. You have the right to an attorney. If you cannot afford an attorney, one will be appointed for you."

Ash remained silent.

Tilson conducted the interrogation. Gibson took notes on a yellow legal pad. However, no recording of the conversation was made by the agents. Tilson asked Ash to show his identification particularly a government issued photo which had his home address. Ash produced his driver's license which he luckily updated after moving to Providence. Satisfied Tilson asked for his social security number which seemed to have matched with the number he had in his possession.

The FBI already knew that Ash purchased a one-way ticket to New Delhi, and he did not have a visa to remain in the U.S.

Ash was impatient and nervous where this interview is leading to. He was unsure why the FBI is questioning him. He looked at Tilson and asked, "Why was I taken off the plane? Why am I being detained?"

Tilson quickly responded to his queries with a query of his own,

"Have you recently made a threat against the president of the United States?"

Ash couldn't believe what he just heard. It was like a bombshell that descended on him. He immediately protested, "No. I made no such threat."

Tilson continued, "We have information leading the FBI to believe that you made a threat to assassinate the president of the United States."

Ash replied in a panic, "What? Where did you get that information from? What is your source?"

No reply was forthcoming from Tilson.

Ash continued, "I am not political. I carry no fire arms. I never owned a gun in my life. What is my motivation to harm the president?" he angrily questioned the agent.

Tilson sniped, "Why are you leaving the country then?"

Ash replied, "It is a long story. The simple reason is my present immigration status. I no longer have valid visa which permits me to remain in the United Status. I am voluntarily returning to my home country to start a new life."

Ash realized that the charges against him are serious and he needed an attorney before he continued the conversation in order to avoid any possible self-incrimination.

He asked the FBI agents, "Am I entitled to make a phone call?"

Tilson replied, "Please feel free. You have a mobile phone on you, don't you?"

Ash reached for his cell phone in his pocket. Ash excused himself and stepped away from the table to make the phone call. He called his older brother Samir in Austin, Texas.

Ash explained to Samir that he has been ejected from his flight home by the FBI agents and is now under detention at the Newark airport. He explained that he is being questioned about an alleged threat he made to kill the American president.

Sam was in disbelief. He immediately concluded that the allegation is totally untrue. He does not have any enemies who would report such an insidious act by him. Someone, possibly his ex-wife planted this untruth. However, he did not share his initial suspicion with Ash.

Sam asked, "How long will you be detained at the Newark airport. Can you find out?"

Ash interrupted his conversation with his brother and turned to Tilson and questioned, "Mr. Tilson, how long will I be detained here?"

Tilson responded, "Not sure. We are awaiting the Secret Service agents. It is up to them to make that decision."

Ash relayed the message he heard from Tilson to Sam. Sam realized without Ash asking that he need to line up a defense attorney to participate in the questioning of his brother by the FBI and Secret Service agents.

He told Ash, "Let me see whether I can have an attorney by your side before you are questioned further. I will be get back to you."

Before clicking off the phone Sam cautioned, "I hope your mobile phone will still stay with you and it will not confiscated by the Federal agents."

Ash returned to the cold metal chair he occupied before and told the FBI agents, "I object to this entire interview. I need my attorney to be present before I can answer further questions from you."

Tilson looked at him. "I understand the complexity involved in getting your attorney down here. You are free to wait until your lawyer shows up, but that will prolong your detention. You may be locked up in a jail such as the Northern State Prison or the Rikers Island jail for days until we can reschedule this interrogation when your lawyer is present. The answers you provide to my questions may cut short your custody. You make the decision."

Ash pondered over the choice Tilson offered. He decided that he does not want to be locked up in a jail until your Sam lined up a lawyer to be by his side when he is questioned by the FBI. That may be days from now. I'll be jeopardizing future charges if I say anything incriminating. He knew he was totally innocent of the charge that is leveled against him. He wanted his detention to end so he can leave their custody.

Ash asked Tilson, "Why is the Secret Service involved in this?"

Tilson replied "A threat against the president of the United States is a federal felony. Under the law a person making a knowing and willful threat shall be fined or imprisoned for no less than five years or both."

Tilson failed to explain that the legal terms of knowing and willful translate to opportunity and intent. Tilson had no obligation to explain the legal terms. The FBI agent remained silent as it is up to the Secret Service to determine the veracity of the perceived threat.

However Tilson was friendly enough to appraise Ash of the gravity of his situation. He continued, "Secret Service special agents will soon be here to conduct an investigation of the threat. We are a Federal Agency who is ensuring that you did not leave the country in light of the threat. We are initiating the questioning to help out the Secret Service. The protocol of the Secret Service is to conduct an interview directly with you, complete an investigation and use their expertise to make a determination."

Ash persisted in his previous question to Tilson and asked, "Can you share with me the source of the information the Secret Service received about the alleged threat?"

Tilson thought for a short while whether to reveal the source. He finally relented and said, "We heard it is Dr. Sara Sharma."

Ash could not believe his ears. He blurted with a passion, "She framed me! Tenacious witch!" Sudden hatred toward Sara filled him like bile.

Tilson realized that he overstepped his authority by revealing the complainer's name. But it was too late. He cannot recant what he already revealed.

Ash looked at his watch. It displayed 11:05 PM. He wondered how much longer he will be detained for questioning. He did not know whether his checked bag was removed from the airplane following his ejection. As he pondered these questions, Tilson's mobile phone rang. Tilson stepped outside the room and answered it. It was Sarkissian on the other end.

"Excuse me," Tilson said before he moved away from the table to take the call.

Sarkissian spoke, "Hi guy, Jim Puller and I just landed at La Guardia. It is 11:10 now. By the time we scoot over to the Newark airport it may be well past midnight. It is getting late for Puller and I. I know it is way, way too late for you as well. I would like to do my interview with the subject in the morning.

"Is there a safe place to hold the subject for the night?" asked Sarkissian.

Tilson replied, "The subject cannot stay at the TSA facilities overnight. I already ascertained it. Where do you suggest we take him for the night?"

Sarkissian replied, "The information that we pieced together preliminarily leads us to believe that the subject could become a problem for ICE to deal with. Is there an ICE Detention Center where he can be sheltered for the night?"

Jim Puller who was doing a Google search for a local ICE Detention Center in New Jersey hollered, "Yes, I found one. It is the Essex County Correctional Facility. It is not too far from the Newark airport."

Tilson heard the holler on his phone.

Sarkissian remarked, "The ICE in Essex County it is! Tilson, please drop off the subject there. We will handle from here on. Please tell the subject we will see him in the morning. Thank you for your immense help with the detention. Your effort was heroic. I appreciate it. You guys are great and a pleasure to work with. Goodbye."

—

Before going to bed that night in a Manhattan hotel room,

Sarkissian once again studied up on the subject's background, digested the enormous amount of data that was gathered on him. Until his detention today, Ash's public record has been clean. He had never been in trouble with the law. Not even a speeding ticket.

Sarkissian wanted to make the subject comfortable enough during the interview so he would open up and reveal something real and true of himself which precipitated his threat. He wanted to have an authentic engagement of some kind with him rather than a stiff interrogation.

—

After answering the phone call Tilson returned to Ash and Bud and announced, "The Secret Service agents have just arrived in New York's La Guardia airport from Washington, D.C. It will take an hour or more for them to get here. Due to the lateness of the night, they decided to meet with you in the morning."

Tilson looked at the subject and said, "You will meet with them at a Newark's Immigration & Customs Enforcement Detention Center. We will drive you to the Center now."

Tilson and Gibson led him to a black Cadillac parked outside the room where he was detained. He did not notice his hand-carry luggage that Gibson wheeled off the airplane. Ash turned to Gibson and queried, "Where is my hand-carry luggage that was removed from the plane? Where is the luggage that I checked in? Has it been taken off the airplane?"

Gibson assured him, "Don't worry. They are in a safe place. You will get them back in due course."

What the FBI agents did not tell Ash is that both bags were being searched for any evidence that may incriminate him in the terrorist threat.

As the Cadillac pulled into the ICE facility, he read a large sign posted in front of a chain-link fence that surrounded the facility. It read Essex County Correctional Facility. It looked like a fortified jail. Two security guards opened the noisy chain-link gate. Tilson identified himself and Gibson sitting on the front seat next to him as FBI agents and told them, "I have a detainee to drop off."

After entering the reception area of the ICE facility, the FBI agents announced they brought in a detainee to drop off. They were handed a bunch of papers attached to a clipboard to fill out. Gibson filled them and returned to the staff. Tilson and Gibson bid Ash goodbye wishing him good luck and started to leave.

Ash remembered that he does not have other clothes to wear than what he is wearing now. He turned to Tilson and asked, "Where is my luggage, Sir? I need my clothes. When can I get it back?" Tilson dismissively replied, "You will get it back!"

—

The ICE staff worker summoned Ash to empty his pockets and the backpack he was carrying on his shoulder into a large see-through zip-lock bag. He took possession of the zip-lock bag, led Ash to an isolated cell and locked the door from outside. The only furniture in the cell was a large wooden bench.

The staff worker addressed him from outside the cell bars, "Sorry, we don't have a jail cell with a bed and a toilet. This facility is completely booked. We use this cell for temporary day-time detention. You need to make do with the bench for the night."

Ash had no other choice than lie down on the cold, hard bench. It was well past midnight. He silently hoped, "*Luckily I will need to spend only a few hours before the night is over. Perhaps tomorrow will be a better day and I may be released.*"

Ash was awakened by noises from other detainees in nearby jail cells who woke up before dawn.

A new staff worker of ICE opened the lock on his cell door and asked, "Do you want to use the facilities? This is your chance."

Before Ash could respond the staff worker announced, "By the way, someone from the Secret Service will see you at 8:30 AM sharp. Be ready."

Ash stood up. He was directed to a nearby large toilet room with facilities including a row of wash basins fitted with running water faucets. He used the toilet and washed his face, rinsed his mouth, combed his hair using his fingers to make himself presentable to the Secret Service agents who will interview him later that morning.

The staff guy ushered him into a large cafeteria-style dining area. He picked up a steel serving tray from the cafeteria line which was filled with a plate of hot meal, fruit and coffee. This was the first meal he had been offered since being ejected from the airplane. Out of necessity he ate the tasteless food and returned to his cell.

It was just before 8:30 in the morning. The ICE staff person came up to the jail cell where Ash was seated and announced, "Hey, your guys from the Secret Service are here. They will meet you in our conference room." He opened the locked door to his cell from outside and led Ash to the conference room.

—

MICHAEL SARKISSIAN AND JAMES Puller were seated in hard wooden chairs resting their arms on chair's arm rests in front of a rectangular table. Sarkissian held out his hand and introduced himself as a special agent of Protective Intelligence in the U.S. Secret Service, followed by introducing Palmer as a fellow agent. Ash was asked to sit across the table from them. It was a wide table.

The conference room is now the Secret Service's interrogation room.

Sarkissian opened the interrogation with this comment, "Mr. Sharma, I believe you know why were taken off the airplane yesterday and detained. The Secret Service received an alert that you made a threat to assassinate the president of the United States. Is it true?"

Before Ash replied he eyed a tape recorder was set up on the table and is recording the conversation. Additionally, Puller opened up a yellow legal pad and started to take notes. He wanted to ask whether an attorney representing him should be present during the questioning but decided it will be a futile request. He did not know whether Samir was able to arrange an attorney to participate in this interview. His brother may not have had time to line up a lawyer given that he was notified of his detention late last night after business hours and it is too early this morning. Ash believed that he is innocent and is not concerned that what he has to say in the interview will incriminate him as he had not committed a crime.

The long silence prompted Sarkissian to set the stage for the conversation. He said, "We are recording our conversation. The recordation should not intimidate you. It is needed only to prepare an accurate report for our records. There are no cameras here. Just a tape recorder! Do I make myself clear?"

Sarkissian maintained eye contact with Ash as he awaited answer.

Ash nodded in agreement. He cleared his throat and finally replied, "No, not true. I am not a political person. I have nothing against the president. I only have admiration for the United States as a country and for American people for their generosity. America is an exceptional country in the world." He looked directly at Sarkissian's blue eyes as he answered.

Even though Sarkissian already knew the answer he gratuitously asked, "Do you carry a gun? Do you have a license to use a weapon to kill?"

"No. I don't' carry a gun or another weapon to kill. I never owned one, never used one and never had to obtain a license for such weapon," emphatically replied Ash.

Sarkissian calibrated his tone and energy level and pelted his next question, "Why are you fleeing the United States? You purchased a one-way ticket out. I understand you held a well-paying job in Providence. What prompted you to abruptly leave the country?"

"I came to this country years ago on a temporary H1B visa from India. My H1B visa expired two months ago. I was under a grace period of sixty days from my visa's expiration date which ended yesterday. I decided to voluntarily leave the U.S. before the grace period expired," answered Ash.

Ash supplemented his answer with, "Sir, I am a law-abiding person. I respect the laws of this country. I felt that leaving the country was the best option under the circumstances."

Sarkissian played dumb and asked, "What do you mean by *the circumstances*?"

Ash responded, "I think you probably know the circumstances I was facing. My wife unexpectedly divorced me a few days ago. She also withdrew the petition she filed with USCIS for my marriage green card. My employer inadvertently failed to renew my H1B visa permit two months ago. Should I say more?"

Ash paused and continued to elaborate, "Mr. Sarkissian, I should have tracked the expiration date of my H1B visa and taken steps to have it renewed, but I failed to do so because of the circumstance of the unexpected divorce by my ex-wife. The divorce stressed me out and distracted me from paying attention to the status of my H1B."

The special agent attentively observed his language style and body language. He sensed a feeling of remorse and regret for the mistake he made in letting his H1B expire.

Sarkissian leaned forward and asked with curiosity, "Do you have any enemies? I mean by that someone who might have framed you to threaten the life of the president?"

Ash became aware from his interview of last night with the FBI agents that his ex-wife is the person who called the Secret Service and falsely alleged that he made the threat. He wondered whether the FBI agents communicated to the Secret Service agents the answers they gathered from the previous night's interview. He wanted to be consistent with what he told the FBI. He wanted to be open and tell his story as he had nothing to hide or be fearful about.

Ash responded with a confident voice, "No. I do not have any enemies. However, I came to know last night from the FBI agents who interviewed me that my former wife is the one who notified the authorities of such a threat. It is a false notification. I never communicated to her of a threat to harm the president. Tell me why would I make such threat since I am dispassionate when it comes to politics?"

"Perhaps you were enraged about her decision to dissolve your marriage. Perhaps the attack on the president is a way to solve the problem of divorce.

"You know divorce is a rejection of love and a traumatic event. It may have triggered the threat of violence in you," said Sarkissian by pounding the table.

"No, not true. I was heart-broken and unhappy with the divorce. However, I do not have a violent streak in me. Please check my record. I was never arrested for any crime, either for a nonviolent crime or a crime involving weapons. I have never been incarcerated. I am a decent and respectable person who minded my career and the well-being of my family," was the passionate outburst from Ash.

Sarkissian looked at his watch. It has been nearly two hours since he started the interview. He stood up to stretch his body.

He announced, "We need a bathroom break."

With those words, the agents pressed the pause button on the taping device and stepped out.

Jim Puller was silent during the entire interview. He could have been a fly on the wall except for notes-taking and monitoring the audio recording equipment.

—

WHILE STANDING AND USING the urinal in the men's restroom, Puller checked for messages on his smart phone. A message received from his buddy at the NSA caught his attention which he quickly read.

Puller took Sarkissian outside to the lawn area away from anyone who can hear what he had to say. He looked at Sarkissian and said, "Mike, this may not be important in our present investigation, but I took the liberty of asking my buddy at the NSA to check on the informant who reported the threat. I had a hunch that she may have falsified the threat. I asked my buddy to investigate her recent associations and travel. Here is what NSA discovered from the GPS location data on her phone. The doctor met with another doctor, Dr. Raj Kumar in Rochester, MN days before she filed for divorce. Also, she and Dr. Kumar went to the same medical school in India and were contemporaries and knew each other."

Puller paused and asked, "Perhaps, the informant and Dr. Kumar conspired to frame the subject of the threat against the president?"

Sarkissian: "Jim, good for taking the lead. I had a similar suspicion about the caller. I wanted to first meet with the subject and then have her investigated if a need arose. You may have jumped the gun, but that is okay. Thanks for this information. I may question the subject on this latest information."

—

AFTER THE SECRET SERVICE AGENTS returned to the conference room and turned on the taping device Sarkissian asked the subject, "How long were you living apart from your wife before the divorce?"

Ash responded, "My employer offered me a new position in Providence about six to seven months ago. My then wife didn't want to move as she was gainfully employed in Ann Arbor. I accepted my new job and moved from Ann Arbor, where my former wife and I lived together, to Providence. She remained in Ann Arbor. Actually, she moved in with her parents who live in that city."

Sarkissian queried, "Has your ex-wife traveled anywhere recently?"

"Yes. She went to Rochester, Minnesota about two months ago. She wanted to meet a classmate from her med school who traveled from India to attend a doctors' conference held at the Mayo Clinic there. I could not join her since I started my new work in Providence."

Ash then remembered that Sara also traveled to India also. He supplemented his answer by saying, "I just remembered this. Before that she traveled to India to attend her class reunion of doctors. The reunion was actually on a cruise ship from India to the Maldives. I could not join her then either because of my work."

Ash waited patiently. There was silence. Ash broke the silence and asked, "I am curious to know why you ask. What relevance does her travel have to the alleged threat?"

Sarkissian hesitated, "Not sure, yet. Do you know the name of the doctor she met in Rochester?"

Ash scratched his head to remember the name, but he couldn't.

He replied, "I don't know. When my ex-wife returned from her trip to Rochester, I recall asking over the phone how her trip went and whether she was able to see her classmate at the conference. She totally ignored my question. Instead, she dropped the bombshell of wanting a divorce."

Sarkissian noticed the details in what he said about his ex-wife's travels. In particular, the detail of her traveling alone without him has registered in Sarkissian's brain.

Sarkissian wanted to jog his memory to recall the name of the doctor she met in Rochester. Ash could not immediately recall the name of her classmate from med school that Sara mentioned in their phone conversation prior to her travel to Rochester.

Ash hesitated and said, "The name is at the tip of my tongue, but I just cannot seem to recall." The tip of his tongue was visible between his lips while Ash tried to recall the name.

Then Sarkissian lost his patience with the subject's recollection of the name. He blurted, "Did she go to meet with Dr. Raj Kumar at the conference in Rochester?"

Ash quickly responded, "That is a man's name. She informed prior to her trip that she was meeting with a female classmate from her med school. Oh! I just remembered. Her classmate's name is Fatima. Are you sure you have the correct name of the doctor she met in Rochester?"

After that remark delivered by the subject, Sarkissian realized that he inadvertently may have opened a Pandora's box created by the ancient Greeks as a punishment to human behavior.

Although he additionally wanted to ask about her travel to Maldives for her class reunion, he decided not to pursue the topic of his ex-wife's travels any further.

Sarkissian's pointed question of, "*Did she go to Rochester to meet with Dr. Raj Kumar*" stuck in Ash's brain and he could not shake it off. He stared at the ceiling of the room.

That question provoked new thoughts and more questions in his head, "*Did Sara have another man in her life? Was he her lover? Was he the reason for Sara to divorce me? Obviously, Sara lied to me when she told him that she was meeting her female classmate Fatima in Rochester,*" he pondered.

The rush of these thoughts bewildered Ash. "*I can't let her get away with this,*" he said to himself. His hands were tight fists on the table. "*I want to bring her down,*" he resolved.

Sarkissian noticed the abrupt change in his subject's mood. He noticed an agitation from his body language.

He reviewed his notes so far. His handwriting was small and beautifully drawn. He put away the pen and the yellow pad. He decided to end the interview.

He said, "I think we will stop this interview for now. If I have any more questions, I will contact you."

Ash nervously queried, "Does this mean I am free to go? Am I free to leave the country and go back to India like I intended before I was ejected from the airplane?"

"No. I am not sure. Those questions will be answered by ICE."

Ash exhaled sharply in disappointment.

Sarkission wanted to appraise Ash on the Secret Service's work on his case. "I will share with you what remains to be completed by the Secret Service Agency. We need to complete the assessment of the threat that was brought to our attention. The information you provided in our interview this morning is helpful to complete the assessment. I wanted to meet you in-person which I am glad I did. If the assessment determines that you are not a threat to the president, then that will be the end of the matter and your case at the Agency will be closed," said Sarkissian.

Those words were music to Ash. With discernible hesitation in his voice Ash asked, "Mr. Sarkissian, may I ask a question."

Ash paused. Sensing that the agent was not objecting, he continued, "Based on your preliminary assessment and the data you gathered on me can you provide me an indication of where I stand in your assessment?"

Sarkissian listened to his question. He did not jump to respond. He wanted to formulate a preliminary assessment from the information on Ash that was gathered so far including the fresh information that he gleaned from the interview he just completed. He applied his past experience of investigating similar cases to the present case.

A person who poses an actual threat does not normally make threats, especially direct threats like the subject was reported to have made. Second, the subject has no mental illness although such illness rarely plays a role in assassination's behavior. Finally, the subject does not fit any one proven descriptive profile of an assassin. He does not seem to have engaged in preparatory decisions and activities to kill the president.

Sarkissian looked the subject directly into his eyes. He said, "This is preliminary! Very preliminary! And don't quote me on this. Do you understand?"

Ash nodded in agreement and said, "Yes."

Sarkissian then calmly stated with a wink, "I don't think you fit the proven profile of an assassin."

With those parting words the Secret Service agents picked up their belongings and left the conference room.

On their way out of the Detention Center Sarkissian told the ICE staff, "The subject is all yours now. We are done interviewing him. He was under a temporary visa which expired. He missed his intended voluntary departure from the country yesterday because the Federal agents detained him for questioning. How you deal with him is now a matter for ICE."

Ash remained in the conference room, which was comfortable compared to the cold and damp bench in the cell where he was locked up before. The ICE staff conferred with his superiors. A decision was reached to handle the subject as a violator of the U.S. immigration laws and be detained for a formal review and adjudication by an immigration judge.

An hour later, the ICE staff member entered the conference room where Ash was seated.

He addressed Ash, "I believe your temporary H1B visa expired. You also exhausted the sixty-day grace period after the H1B expired. You are in violation of the U.S. immigration laws. An immigration judge will need to review your case. Until then you will be a detained by ICE."

Ash tried to protest, "I believe my visa expired yesterday. I was set to voluntarily leave the country before my visa expired, but last night I was forcibly detained by the FBI for questioning. Technically I did not violate the immigration law since I was ready, willing and able to depart the country yesterday."

Ash's protest was ignored by the staff. Instead, he questioned Ash, "Does your family live in the Newark- New York area? This Center is completely booked with other detainees. We have no room to keep you here. ICE will move you to another Center which is convenient to your family members for possible visitation while you are in detention."

"I do not have family in this area. I have a brother who lives in Austin, Texas," replied Ash.

The ICE staff member left the room for almost an hour leaving Ash alone. When he returned, he carried the transparent zip-lock bag where Ash's backpack and contents were stored the night before.

He said, "I have good news for you. The Central Texas Detention Center in San Antonio is the place where you will be detained. A military plane that is scheduled to go to San Antonia will take you there. The plane will depart in three hours."

—

THE NEXT THING THAT HAPPENED was Ash and four other detainees and an armed guard were driven to the McGuire Air Force Base in New Jersey and put on a C-130 plane loaded with heavy military cargo. A military crew member on the plane confirmed to the guard that the plane is destined for San Antonia, Texas.

They got on the plane and sat on what looked like jump seats that flight attendants normally occupy in commercial flights during takeoff and landing. The C-130 was loaded with max-armored vehicles chained next to the jump seat that Ash occupied.

CHAPTER 12

ASH GOT OFF THE MILITARY PLANE that brought him from Newark to San Antonio. As the ICE's security guard drove him and his fellow detainees, Ash's mobile phone vibrated in his pocket. He answered. It was his brother Sam from Austin.

"Hi, I have been calling you, but you did not answer. I am glad that you answered now. What is going on?" Sam queried.

Ash told him, "I am under ICE custody now and am being transported to the Central Texas Detention Facility in San Antonia."

He could not discuss anything about his interviews with the FBI and the Secret Service agents who decided to move him to the custody of ICE because the guard was listening to his conversation.

Ash told his brother, "Sam, please contact me at the Detention Center in San Antonio tomorrow," and silenced his phone.

The Texas facility was immense with a chain-link fence and barbed wire atop the fence surrounding it like the Essex facility he left earlier this afternoon. The difference Ash noticed was that in addition to the high-rise permanent structures a few prefabricated white tents were erected on the vast grounds. As the van drove into the facility Ash could see it was eerily quiet except for some human activity around the tents.

A large sign in front of the main building read: Immigration and Customs Enforcement Detention Facility, Department of Homeland Security (DHS), Managed by the GEO Group Inc. (Private and For-Profit).

The van dropped off the detainees in front of the main building and they were directed to the reception area. One by one each detainee went through a metal scan, followed by a pat-down in search of weapons.

In the secure area an ICE officer stood. He loudly announced, "You will be asked to provide us information about your name, address, social security number if you have one, and identify your relatives who might visit you at this facility." He added the warning, "Any statement you make may be used against you in a subsequent proceeding."

After that the ICE officer asked the newly arrived group to fill out the paperwork which he handed out attached to a clipboard.

One of the questions in the requested paper was, "Why are you being detained?"

Ash was stumped by this request, particularly in light of the warning the officer just gave. Ash exhaled. He wanted to be truthful in his statement. He told himself he had not done anything wrong and the truth will prevail.

He gasped in frustration and wrote down the response, "Yesterday was the last day of my valid H1B visa. I was aboard a flight bound for India to voluntarily leave the U.S. before my visa expired. I was forcibly ejected from my flight by the Secret Service to question about an alleged threat I made to harm the president of the U.S. I made so such threat. After questioning me, I was handed over to ICE today for continued custody."

The ICE officer perused what Ash wrote. His reaction was, "Wow! A threat of terrorism! This is a felony and pretty serious stuff. I tell you, this seems like mandatory detention to me. The immigration judge will not be able to grant you bail. You may need an attorney to get you out, my friend."

The officer's gratuitous comment alarmed Ash. He wanted to protest that he is innocent and should not even be detained but realized that is futile as the officer is not the person who will judge his innocence or guilt.

Ash was assigned a file number beginning with a capitalized first letter of the English alphabet. It was: A-3943. He was told to use the A-number in all communications including for visitation by family, friends and the attorney who may represent him.

He announced, "Social and family visits between 12 PM and 9 PM. Attorney visits between 9 AM to 9 PM. Remember, only two visitors at a time!"

The officer confiscated Ash's cell phone and the backpack he was carrying telling him that he will get these back when he is finally released from the Facility.

Ash was sent to a prison cell inside the main high-rise. The cell was designed for use by two people as there were two beds stacked one on top of another. He knew a cell mate might join him. Since the cell was not occupied, he decided to use the lower bed.

He stretched out on the bed and wondered how long he will be detained there and what battles with law enforcement that lay ahead for him.

An ICE officer came by his prison cell. He announced, "Your brother tracked you down at our Facility. He wishes to meet with you. The visitation is scheduled for tomorrow at noon. Go to the visitation area to meet him. Your visitation should be limited to twenty minutes. Okay?" and left.

Ash's thoughts shifted to the many events in his life that have gone differently and how quickly he lost control over them and ended up in his present situation. He reflected on his past year of life with Sara and the series of events that took place. He came to the conclusion that Sara planned everything. She unilaterally decided to petition for his marriage green card. She abruptly decided to divorce him. She withdrew the petition for his green card. After the divorce was finalized, she reported a concocted plot by him to assassinate the president. All of these events were planned by Sara right down to the last detail.

Ash thought some more. The missing piece in his puzzle is Sara's motive. Ash wondered, "*Perhaps the reason for her travel to Maldives and Rochester might shed light on her motive. The revelation that she might have met with Dr. Raj Kumar in Rochester may have the clue for her motive. Did she travel to Maldives also to meet Raj?*"

Ash decided that when he is freed from his detention, he will explore the possible relationship between Sara and Raj.

Sara tricked him to sponsor his marriage green card and pulled the plug on it by forcing the divorce. Because he believed he will receive his green card through her sponsorship, Ash neglected to track the status of his H1B visa. The expiration of his H1B forced him to voluntarily leave the country without causing trouble to his employer and to safeguard his re-entry at a future date. His planned departure was interrupted because Sara reported a concocted terrorist plan by him.

It did not take a rocket scientist to figure out Sara's motives. "*Banish Ash from her life so she can start a new life, perhaps with Raj was the inevitable conclusion,*" Ash reached for now.

Ash also wondered whether Sara became psychotic to have her marriage annulled. Did her psychosis lead to her insidious thought of a plot by him to kill the president?

The solitude of the fortress of the prison Ash was locked up did not bother him at first. It offered time to think without disruption and silently strategize his plan of action.

Ash has been an excellent strategist whether in a chess match, solving a mathematical problem or designing complex software architecture to solve business problems. His strategy before solving a problem has been to first bring it to light by gathering facts and know the boundary conditions. Then lay the road to solve it and accept the road. Be prepared to accept the darkest sides of the road and the steepest hill to climb to reach his quest.

The Facility offered Ash the freedom to walk around at permitted times. He wanted to understand the rules and the bureaucracy practiced by ICE so he can devise a plan for release from their custody.

He chatted up with other detainees and observed their behavior. But being confined to a pit with little opportunity for genuine intellectual stimulation drove him crazy.

On his second night at the Facility as Ash was beginning to fall asleep in his bed the rattle of an ICE officer opening the door of his prison cell awakened him.

"You have a cellmate now," the officer announced and let in a middle-aged, brown-skinned man into the jail cell. He was about five feet tall and displayed moderate muscles in his arms and chest. The officer locked up the cell's door and left.

Ash introduced, "Hi, I am Ash. I arrived yesterday."

The man stretched out to shake Ash's hand saying, "I am Hugo." Ash shook his hand. His hand was hard and rough with callouses that he could feel as he shook indicating that he used his hands for tough and hard work.

Hugo looked around and realized that the upper bed is his to use.

"Amigo, I have been around for a couple of weeks now. They decided to move me from another section of the prison to this cell now," continued Hugo.

"Amigo, what are you being detained for?" asked Hugo as he climbed to his bed.

Ash gave him a quick rundown of what transpired in the last two days.

He said, "I was voluntarily leaving the U.S. two nights ago. They detained me from leaving. It looks like I am being held on a terrorism charge which is completely false."

"Amigo, you don't look like a terrorist to me. You look like a fine college boy," remarked Hugo.

"What are you here for?" asked Ash looking up from his bed.

"Not sure. I was originally detained for deportation for illegally entering the U.S. Then the charge was upped to possession and illegal sale of drugs in Texas. They say my custody status is now mandatory detention. I am not sure what the hell is going on," said Hugo.

—

ASH MET WITH HIS BROTHER the next day as scheduled. After greeting each other, the brothers quickly got down to brass tags. Ash took Sam through the ordeal he faced with the FBI and Secret Service agents in Newark. Sam was gratified that the Secret Service preliminarily concluded that his brother did not fit the profile of a terrorist, but he was troubled that ICE is holding him on terrorism related grounds. Dismissal of Ash's case by the immigration judge may not be easy unless he is represented by an experienced attorney who can pull together the evidence and convince DHS and the judge for dismissal.

Sam related, "I will line up an experienced counselor from a San Antonio law firm to represent you Ash. It will take a few days as I must talk to friends and relatives who can help me identify such a lawyer. I need to negotiate the terms with him. Good and reputable immigration lawyer charge high fees. But money is not a consideration. I want you out of the detention facility as soon as possible."

The twenty minutes of Sam's visit was ending, and he was getting ready to leave his brother. Ash intercepted, "Sam, What I am going to say is not urgent, but I want to share my thoughts on this. I am prohibited from access to email or the internet. When I have access to a computer, I would like to check up on Dr. Raj Kumar. Sara saw him in Rochester two months ago. Raj apparently was Sara's contemporary at Osmania Medical School. I would like to check whether Sara met with Raj when she went for her class reunion on the cruise from India to Maldives. I have a suspicion that they together conspired to end my marriage which led Sara to launch the divorce action, withdraw my marriage green card and then falsely report the terrorist threat."

Sami agreed and replied, "Ash, I can help you with that. First things first, I want to get you out of this jail."

—

ASH FOUND HIS CELLMATE Hugo very resourceful. He relayed to him his life history of being born to an agricultural farmer in the southern Mexican state of Chiapas bordering with Guatemala. His father insisted on his son to go to school and receive good education. Hugo held jobs from his early teen years doing whatever job he could find while attending school to earn money. He was of help to butchers, gun makers, blacksmiths and smugglers who smuggled goods and people in and out of Mexico across the border with Guatemala. He has been married and has four children who live close to his parents' house. His family depended on him for money to survive.

Hugo bragged he had done many jobs in his life in many countries including commissioning coyotes to smuggle drugs and people across borders. He sounded confident in what he said, as Ash suspected about Hugo's past deeds.

Ash did not ask how he ended up getting caught by law enforcement, but Hugo was knowledgeable of the criminal world and how it worked. Without asking Ash knew that Hugo had brush with law enforcement before and he was astute enough about the law enforcement system in the U.S., Mexico, Guatemala and other countries to be able to get around them.

Hugo was friendly to talk with, addressing him always as Amigo. Ash soon established a good rapport with him to talk about the detention Facility and to share his inner thoughts and feelings.

—

THE FACILITY HOUSED YOUNG MEN and women between eighteen and forty-five years. The women were separated from the men by a chain-link fence and housed in separate quarters. The men and women were drawn from all over the world, but the majority came from the southern and Central American countries including Mexico, Guatemala, El Salvador and Honduras. Ash saw some from Bangladesh, China, India, Pakistan and Vietnam. He could guess their country of origin from their skin color, facial features and the language they spoke.

The detainees included drug smugglers, human traffickers and people who crossed the U.S. border without a valid visa and other violators of U.S. immigration laws. They were sent to the Facility to adjudicate their case before an immigration judge. Ash learned that depending on the complexity of the case and the judge's docket load, the adjudication may take as little time as a week to several months.

—

SAM LINED UP AN EXPERIENCED immigration lawyer from San Antonia and brought him to the Detention Facility to introduce him. The lawyer is Matt Miller. Ash shook hands with Miller as they took seats in the visitation area of the Facility. The lawyer looked polished with a bow tie attached to a white-collar shirt matching the suit he wore. He appeared to be in his mid-to-early forties.

Miller explained that he has handled many court cases that came up for adjudication before immigration judges. He has a track record of success in most of them over his twenty years of experience.

"Mr. Sharma, I must tell you what you see at this Facility is an assembly line adjudication process where a large number of cases of individuals seeking protection from deportation are commingled with others who are willing, like you, to leave the country voluntarily. As a result the court's docket is overloaded and the judge is pressured to render quick determinations on cases and manage the load from growing and overwhelming the docket."

Miller paused, looked around and added, "I know a couple of the immigration judges. Knowing the judge is a great help to resolve an immigration case before that judge."

With that Ash decided to engage Miller to represent him, politely asking him, "Can we drop the Mister stuff? Address me simply as Ash."

Miller advised, "Ash, whatever you tell me is protected by the rules of attorney-client privilege. So, please tell me the full details without fear of breach of confidentiality or self-incrimination. I need to know the truth to be able to defend you. Do you understand?"

Ash said, "I understand." He narrated his story in excruciating detail as Miller took notes on a large yellow legal pad. Miller seldom interrupted him. He quietly listened as his mind worked on a solution to handle Ash's case based on what he heard from his client.

Miller stopped taking notes and looked at Ash and Samir expecting question from them.

Ash asked, "What is the quickest way to obtain a release so I can go back to India?" Second, "Am I eligible for release by posting bail while my case is pending for resolution?"

"Let me address your second question first. Whether you are eligible for release by posting a bond? Unfortunately, your case is caught in the bureaucracy of DHS. You were incorrectly classified as a terrorism-related case when it should have been listed as voluntary departure after visa expiration. Because of this mix-up your detention is a mandatory custody instead of a general custody and you are ineligible for release by posting a bond."

Miller continued, "Two facts are working against you to seek a bail. First the Secret Service is now investigating your threat against the life of the president which is a felony. Second, the agency ejected you from a flight out of the country. The ejection proved you are a flight risk. The immigration judge will not release you on your own recognizance, I am afraid."

"I have a strategy to obtain your release," continued Miller by looking at Ash. "This is my strategy."

Miller paused as Ash and Samir looked at him anxiously.

"I will obtain from the Secret Service the final report on their threat investigation. I am hoping it will say that the alleged threat is unfounded and you have no history of violence or crimes committed, no gun ownership, not mentally ill and you do not fit the profile of a terrorist. Once I obtain that report, I will file an application for relief to the immigration judge that you should be allowed to leave the country voluntarily."

"I will try to speed up your release, but it depends on how quickly I can obtain the report from Secret Service and determine what it says. That report will be the key to the court's deliberations. It also depends on how quickly I have an individual hearing scheduled with the judge and the Counsel of DHS where the merits of the case will be presented by the two opposing counsels."

"In the meanwhile, I am afraid you will continue to be detained here," declared Miller.

"I have already been in this detention Facility for more than a week. Can you appraise me on the expected date for the hearing?" asked Ash as Miller got ready to leave the premises.

"I can't tell you that Ash. I'll do my best to speed up the hearing," said Miller. He waived his hand and said, "Good bye. Have a good weekend, if that is possible!"

—

WHILE ON IMMIGRATION HOLD, Ash continued chatting with Hugo. Their mutual comradery grew to a comfortable level of trust to talk about various issues that are on their minds. The open grounds near the tents offered opportunities to talk as they observed other inmates.

Hugo pointed to a flea-infested vagrant at a distance, "Look at this vagrant. I have been watching him. He is disgusting. He refuses to wash, refuses to have a bath and smells. When he scratches his head, I wouldn't want to know what comes out."

Ash bemoaned to Hugo, "My ex-wife planned the events which caused my detention and the hardship I have been facing in my life. I loved her and trusted her. Unbeknownst to me she took control over my life and put me in the situation I am in now."

Hugo asked, "What do you want to do about it? Are you going to look back and feel sorry for yourself or do something?"

Ash "What do you mean? Take retribution?"

"Yes. Something like that," Hugo replied.

"I cannot let my former wife get away with the stress and harm she caused me. She damaged my family's reputation. I am not normally vindictive, but what my ex did is so egregious that I must retaliate," Ash responded with frustration in his voice.

Hugo replied, "Guess what Amigo? I can put you in touch with a person who might help in your cause, whatever that might be. I don't want to hear about your plan, but this guy is someone you may want to use. You can count on him. He will fulfill what he promises."

When they returned to their cell Hugo pulled out a small black book from under his pillow and gave Ash the particulars of Alexis Victor.

Hugo told him, "Victor is an American. I worked with Victor in Guatemala and Mexico. He is good at what he does."

—

THE FOLLOWING MONDAY MILLER called Mike Sarkisssian, the Protective Intelligence Officer at the Secret Service Agency that Ash identified. Miller introduced himself saying, "I am an attorney representing Ash

Sharma in a mandatory detention proceeding before an immigration judge in Central Texas Detention Facility. Miller queried, "Has a decision been reached on the alleged threat of my client to harm the president of the United States?"

Sarkissian responded, "No. Not yet. The evaluation of the threat is nearly complete. However, a final decision has not yet been made. Mr. Miller, It may take more time to reach the decision."

Miller elaborated, "My client has been incarcerated at the ICE Detention Facility for more than two weeks. He was on a flight to voluntarily depart the U.S. before the expiration of his visa. U.S. Secret Service ejected him from the plane and detained him. Because of that detention, *and only because of that detention I must add,* his visa has now expired, and he ended up in the ICE Facility."

Miller continued, "Obviously, my client is eager to get out of the jail and leave the country, but that will happen only if the immigration judge will grant such relief. What is holding up the relief is U. S. Secret Service's determination that my client does not pose a risk to the president."

Sarkissian replied, "I fully understand the situation that your client is facing. Based on my evaluation I can tell you this. There is no proven truth that your client made the threat. He is not mentally ill, has no history of violence or committed crimes, no gun ownership, no motive to harm the president. The records indicate he never posed clear and present danger to anyone."

Miller pressingly asked, "Then, what is holding up your final decision?"

Sarkissian whispered, "It is an internal matter."

Miller asked, "Is it possible to send me a letter stating what you just orally conveyed about my client?"

Miller applied pressure by additionally saying "Or shall I exercise the Freedom of Information Act to have you supply your evaluation under a secrecy order to the immigration judge for deliberation?"

Sarkissian went silent for a minute pondering how to respond. His gut told him that Ash is innocent of the alleged threat. The record of data he gathered on him proves it. Also, under the FOIA his agency will be obligated to share the report to the immigration judge.

He spoke up, "Mr. Miller, yes I am willing to send you such a letter. I hope it will serve as evidence to obtain the relief."

—

THE WHEELS OF JUSTICE turn slowly. It took a week for Miller to receive the letter promised by Sarkissian.

Miller reviewed the letter and was satisfied with its contents. He requested a merits hearing with an immigration judge that he knew from his past dealings. After matching the availability of the judge, the DHS counsel and Miller's own calendar a date was set for a hearing. It was ten business days from now.

Miller met with Ash at the detention Facility again. He appraised him on the progress he was able to make in his case. He collected from his client documents which were confiscated by ICE including his passport, the H1B visa document with its expiration date, the boarding pass issued by United Airlines on the day of his ejection.

Miller advised him to be ready and prepared to participate in the hearing by giving a few useful tips like, "Wear clean and comfortable clothes. Shave your face, comb your hair and present yourself well."

—

THE MERITS HEARING BEFORE the immigration judge took place as scheduled. Only four people participated in the hearing: the presiding judge, the Assistant Chief Counsel of DHS, Miller and Ash. Neither Miller nor the DHS counsel had a co-counsel.

The judge in a black robe and gravel in hand. He was short five feet three. His eyes were dark, gray hair swept back into ponytail and with rimless glasses. The DHS counsel was around fifty but could pass up for forty. He was tanned and wore a gray suit with a white shirt and purple necktie.

Miller was impeccably dressed in a dark blue high-quality suit and his characteristic bow tie on a light blue collared shirt.

The merits of the case were simple. Miller already briefed the opposing counsel and the presiding judge in his private chambers before the formal hearing.

The opening statement was a standard fare. The DHS counsel outlined the charges against the detainee. Miller ignored the charges and dived to defend his client. Miller stood up in front of the judge. He adjusted his bow tie and presented the merits of the case using short sentences in a voice filled with humility and respectfulness.

Miller pleaded, "Your Honor, my client is not guilty of any of the charges that my opposing counsel read. He should be freed from custody and allowed to voluntarily depart the country."

He furnished the document received from the Secret Service Agency and continued his pleading, "The threat to harm the president of the United States is totally unfounded. He has no history of violence or any record of past crimes. He is a law-abiding person. He never even received a traffic ticket. That's how clean his record is."

Miller then produced the evidence of his client's boarding pass, passport and the visa data stamped in it and stated, "The respondent Mr. Sharma was ready, willing and able to leave the country before his valid non-immigration H1B visa expired. The Secret Service ejected him from the plane and detained him. Because of that detention and only because of that detention his visa has now expired, and he ended up in this detention Facility."

The DHS counsel did not call any witnesses. He did not contest the evidence presented by Miller.

With no contest by the opposing counsel the hearing essentially ended. The judge rendered an oral pronouncement of his agreement with Miller's pleading and granted the relief requested.

The judge turned toward Ash and said, "Your voluntary deportation is good for thirty days starting from today" and using his right hand banged the wooden gavel on its sound block with a thunderous sound emphasizing his decision. The court room went quiet.

Outside the court room Miller congratulated his client. He added, "Ash, I did my best to accelerate this outcome. I am sorry that you were detained in this prison for six weeks or may be longer. You certainly did not deserve it. You are free to go home now. By the way, after leaving the country under the law you cannot reenter for a period of ten years." He shook hands with him, gave a hug and left wishing him well.

—

Ash bid adieu to Hugo telling him, "I know you will not stay here too long. You are a clever man and you kept me from going insane. I thank you. Good luck in what you will do after you leave. If I may give you some advice, you should go home and take care of your family. After all, the legacy you leave behind after you are gone is your wife and children."

—

Sam picked his brother up the same evening to take him home to his family in Austin. Before leaving the Facility Ash inquired the ICE staff about his luggage that the FBI confiscated in Newark International airport. The staff shrugged his shoulder saying, "Sorry, I don't know anything about your luggage!"

Ash and Sam concluded that the luggage seems to have mysteriously disappeared.

While Sam was driving his brother to Austin, Ash asked, "Did you have a chance to get any information about Raj and Sara about their meeting in Rochester?"

Sam responded, "No, I have not been able to dig into it. My advice to you Ash is to forget about your past marriage. The sad chapter with your former wife is now closed. Let it go. Focus on your future. Perhaps you can help mom and dad to manage the farmlands they own in Hyderabad. That will be a productive activity and may lead you to calmer existence."

—

ASH CALLED THE UNITED AIRLINES to rebook his one-way ticket from Newark to New Delhi, the flight he was ejected from less than two months ago. He wanted a nonstop international flight. He asked the reservations agent, "Whether United would be able to reinstate the ticket he paid for. "

The agent rejected Ash's request saying, "Sir, you purchased a non-refundable ticket. It cannot be refunded or reissued."

Ash explained the circumstances of his forced ejection, "I was forcibly ejected by the FBI to question me on a charge that was filed against me. That charge has now been proven to be false," he said. He narrated the story following his ejection and the detention. The agent sympathized with the ordeal that Ash went through. He took upon himself to check with his supervisor.

Minutes later he returned and responded to Ash' request, "You have been a loyal customer of United. We appreciate your loyalty. I am glad to tell you that my supervisor agreed to reinstate your canceled ticket. However, we cannot upgrade you this time as our business class is fully booked on the day of your flight."

Ash thanked the United Airlines agent for his generosity. Before he disconnected the phone, Ash casually asked whether United knows what happened to the suitcase he checked on his previous flight. The agent asked him to wait and explored the status of the checked bag.

He returned to the phone and said, "We have two pieces of luggage tagged in your name. They are being held as abandoned property with our Baggage Claims in Newark Airport. Please pick them up at your convenience."

—

Ash's anger toward Sara would not cool down. Ash tried to be optimistic and let go of his unhappiness in his marriage towards the end and the bitterness of divorce, like Sam advised. However, Sara's manipulation of the Secret Service to harass him by cooking up a false story enraged him beyond anything he experienced in his life. The harsh lock up at the detention center and the suffering he endured for six weeks was demeaning and humiliating. She is now the villain in his life as she also restricted his freedom. He vowed revenge.

He vowed, "*She started it, I'll finish it!*"

He decided the fight he will wager against Sara is going to be a under an eye for an eye and a tooth for a tooth kind of tenet.

Ash called his attorney Miller to thank him again for getting him out of the detention Facility. More importantly, Ash wanted to explore legally available retributions against his ex-wife. He asked, "Mr. Miller what legal actions against my ex-wife are available to me as a victim of a false accusation?"

Miller lectured him, "Ash, there are several. All of these are civil actions, which mean you are entitled to money damages only. You cannot file criminal charges against her. The legal recourse you have because you were falsely accused of a crime is a claim of defamation, malicious prosecution or false imprisonment."

Miller paused and continued to elaborate, "First you need proof that you have been exonerated by the Secret Service Agency which means we need to obtain the final report from the Agency. The report must conclude that you did not make a threat against the president and your ex-wife falsely reported such threat. Remember, I tried to obtain this report for your detention hearing, but the Agency did not finalize the report then. I can try to get the report from the Agency again.

"I can file a defamation suit against your ex-wife charging her that she libeled and slandered you. We need to show that she made the statement that you threatened to kill the president and the statement was false. Additionally, we need to show damage to your reputation," stated Miller.

"I can also file a claim against her for intentional tort of malicious prosecution," Miller said in conclusion.

Ash responded, "I want retribution. I have been horribly victimized."

"I understand how you feel. However, all of these claims will take time to prosecute. Time for gathering evidence, filing the complaint, and eventually prove in a court of law. Unfortunately, your tenure in the county is now limited to less than – what - thirty days? Also you cannot reenter the country for ten years. The system of justice even in an advanced country like the United States grinds slowly. I am afraid you do not have the time. Without your physical presence in the country, it will be futile to file these legal claims," were the final words from Miller.

Ash concluded that Miller slammed the final nail in the coffin for launching a legal action against his former wife.

The following morning Ash contacted Alexis Victor.

CHAPTER

13

ASH RETURNED TO HYDERABAD to his parents' home. His room in the house remained the way he left nearly eight years ago. The bookshelves were filled with books from his school and college days. Framed certificates he was awarded for winning essay competitions and degree certificates hung from nails on the walls. Trophies he won in chess matches decorated the shelves. Chess boards and matching chess pieces lay still on the credenza.

"*Those were the good old days. Life was simple and full of hope,*" recalled Ash as he looked around his childhood room. The contents of his room reminded him of his early experiences in life. He remembered of his early experience to strategize while playing chess with his father.

His life in America was truncated by trumped-up charges by his ex-wife. He was subject to confinement in a fortress of solitude for nearly two months because of Sara's grotesque and extreme behavior.

His name was placed on the notorious terrorist list because of her false allegation to the Secret Service.

The physical stress and emotional distress he endured and the humiliation that his family suffered was unforgiving to Ash. Controlling his life by duping him to obtain his green card through her dubious sponsorship and subsequently killing it have put Ash in a legal bind which was beyond any human being could have undertaken, far less by the person who married him and agreed to love him and take care of him in health and in sickness. He concluded Sara turned into an avatar of hellishness.

He lay on his bed undaunted by the hell he went through. For Ash courage and keeping a clear head were not optional, but rather saving virtues of his dignity and reputation. He felt tormented day and night for months. He was suffering. Sara haunted him.

He resorted to brutal tenets rather than forgetting his former wife like his brother advised.

Ash began to strategize a logical game plan of revenge to destroy Sara's life. He vowed that, "*For every day he spent in the ICE Detention Facility, Sara must spend a year in solitude and suffer as a fitting penitence for the ordeal she put him through.*"

First Ash wanted to gather intelligence on Raj and find out how deep was his association with Sara. The Medical School at Osmania was helpful to provide information about their former graduates. He gathered that Raj was a year senior to Sara, but for some reason they both graduated in the same year.

He gathered that Fatima, who attended his wedding, is now a practicing doctor in Dacca.

Ash checked up the Facebook pages of all three classmates. It netted little information from the pages of Raj and Sara, but Fatima was active in posting her activities with friends and family on her Facebook page. She posted several photos of her class reunion taken on the cruise ship which showed Raj and Sara together as a pair along with the group pictures of other classmates and their spouses.

This posting confirmed Ash's suspicion that Sara became reacquainted with Raj at their class reunion.

He now became more convinced that re-acquaintance on the cruise ship was a prelude to Sara meeting with Raj again in Rochester days before she decided to divorce him.

Ash wanted to dig more into a private relationship between Sara and Raj when they lived in the dorms at Osmania. He commissioned a private investigator who is a retired agent of the Central Bureau of Investigation.

He assigned the agent with a specific and limited task of identifying any social or romantic relationship between Sara and Raj when they were in the med school.

The CBI agent was down to earth and practical in his approach. He found out that Raj was an avid tennis player in med school. He inquired from the tennis court attendants whether any females watched Raj while he played tennis. That inquiry did not yield any result.

He then cleverly targeted the dorm cooks at Osmania who prepared special foods at the student's requests, especially when such requests were made late in the night. The report furnished by the investigator revealed that on several occasions Raj and Sara went to the dorm's cafeteria past mid night, some as late at 2 AM. The late night attending cook confirmed that the romantic couple requested him to prepare light snacks and hot chai for them.

A specific comment by the late night cook was, "It is kind of odd that this couple was the only couple who frequented late at night and ordered snacks. Invariably, they were not dressed in street clothes, but in night attire."

The CBI reported his conclusion to of some sort of romantic activity between Raj and Sara when they were in med school.

Ash now became more fully convinced that Sara had a romantic relationship with Raj before her marriage. Ash's target for revenge continued to be his ex-wife and not Raj despite the suspected prior romantic relationship between the two. He only could see the negatives in Sara's humanity.

Ash kept up with his purposeful stride.

—

HAVING BEEN SENSITIZED by his name entering the U.S. terrorist list and the surreptitious way intelligence is gathered by NSA, FBI and other U.S. agencies, Ash wanted to mitigate the monitoring of his phone calls with Victor by American intelligence. He purchased used mobile phones and prepaid cell phones for conversing with Victor.

Ash followed up on his introductory call he placed to Victor when he was in Austin.

"Hello Victor. This is Ashwin. I am calling from India like I promised a couple of months ago. Do you remember our brief conversation when I called you from Austin?" he asked.

Victor recognized his earlier contact and acknowledged, "Hello Ashwin, nice to hear from you. Of course I remember our conversation."

Ash continued, "Like I mentioned before, I have a specific mission in mind for you. But I need to know more about you. Can you tell me things about you? Your past work, capabilities, etc.?"

Victor responded, "Yes. I have been with the U.S. Army for twenty years. I am specialized in disposing chemical weapons. Most recently I was sent to Syria by President Trump to inspect chemical weapons that Syria's President Assad used against the Kurds in Northern Iraq. This is dangerous work more than any task that you may have in your mind."

Ash responded, "Yes, for sure!"

Victor continued, "Before that I was assigned for investigate the Iranian government against concealment of nuclear materials like enriched uranium used in making nuclear weapons. I worked with the International Atomic Energy Agency in that tricky mission on the pretext of Iran's noncompliance with certain international agreements."

Victor elaborated, "I am a chemist. All of my prior jobs are related to deploying, detecting and destroying chemical weapons during wars. My previous jobs have been of extremely high risk and deadly."

"Since I retired from the Army about three years ago, I have been a private investigator and handling specific tasks as a hired gun. I am well trained in killing. I am regarded as a professional hit man and a paid assassin," Victor offered as his additional credentials.

Victor the added this, "I am a hacker of computers and computer networks. Through hacking I gather emails and data stored in the cloud."

"Do you execute you mission yourself or depend on others?" asked Ash.

"It depends on the complexity of the mission. I have a network of people that I rely on depending on the mission at hand. I have access to former KGB agents currently residing in the U.S. and people who once worked for the Scotland Yard and many others," was Victor's sharp reply.

Victor paused and continued, "I depend on others in my network for sophisticated computer hacking. For example, to decrypt software codes employed in highly protected computer systems through sophisticated encryption techniques."

Victor pressed Ash, "Please tell me what is on your mind? Is it merely investigative work and gather intelligence on a particular person or is it a mission? If it is a mission, is it serious work to harm somebody? Or is it more serious like an assassination?"

Victor paused and continued, "Remember I am rewarded for my work. I kick some ass. I turn over rocks to find evidence. I use force. I do kidnapping. I do murders. I do counter-terrorism. My commission depends on the nature of what I am asked to do."

Ash hesitated. He was not ready to discuss Victor's fees. He hadn't made up his mind what action he planned and how soon.

He responded somewhat ambiguously, "It first involves investigative work to track a target and get familiar with the target's daily modus operandi. The serious work you referred to will follow depending on what I discover."

Victor added to give Ash confidence in his work. He said, "I may be retired but am current in the investigative game. I am well connected to law enforcement that sometimes those connections are very useful."

Ash asked, "Victor, I would like to know how trust-worthy you are to keep my personal identity and the mission secretive and never disclose it to anyone. I want absolute anonymity and do not wish to be charged with a conspiracy if unfortunately you were to get caught by law enforcement."

Victor responded, "Ash, you can trust me one hundred percent. Your protection is paramount to me. I keep my mouth shut. If I cannot safeguard the identity of my client and the mission, believe me I will not be in my line of business. I cease to exist."

Ash finally said, "Victor, before we go any further, let me digest what you told me. I will get back to you in due course. Okay?" They disconnected their phones.

—

Ash managed to line up an offshore job which needed him to work for home. An India-based recruiter put Ash in touch with CVS Pharmacy which was seeking to fill a position for a computer architect to design and develop a user-friendly computer platform for use by the general public to place online orders for purchase of prescription medicines. Ash's prior years of work experience with Microsoft and Fidelity was an easy sell to get hired for his new job. His new job was well-paying, and his salary paid in U.S. dollars which Ash wanted in order to pay Victor.

Ash worked in real time, which meant working during the night hours because of the over half-a-day time difference between the U.S. and India. His work hours were dictated so he can interact in real time through voice and video conferences with CVS' workers based in the U.S.

—

Unbeknownst to Ash, Sara's life perked up after her divorce and the false report she filed with the Secret Service of a terrorist threat by Ash. She did not know what happened to Ash. She assumed that he has been locked up in a federal penitentiary for the threat against the president. She assumed that her plan worked and Ash is out of her life forever. She had no regrets and showed no remorse for what she had done to Ash and behaved like everything is normal now.

Sara felt that she is open to rejuvenate the past romance she had with Raj. She regularly called Raj to rekindle their past romance. She cooed sweet nothings into his ear to sexually excite him. Sara fantasized a romantic life with him in due course.

Kailash and Sunil Nair were amenable to have their daughter married again. They were pleased that Sara is finally able to remarry, this time a person of her real choice. Kailash told himself "*this time Sara's marriage with Raj is bound to work; and he will be blessed with a grandchild.*"

Sara wanted a destination wedding with Raj. The destination she selected is the Fairmont Banff Springs Hotel in the Canadian Rocky

Mountains. She participated as a bridesmaid in the wedding of her best friend and classmate at Pioneer High School there and loved its spectacular setting.

She dreamed of celebrating her own wedding there, but to her disappointment her father arranged her wedding with Ash in Hyderabad. She felt good that she now has a second chance to have her wedding take place with the love of her choice in her dream location.

The Fairmont hotel is a dream location for sure. The hotel is located in the Banff National Park at an altitude of 4,600 feet and looked over a valley. The property is bounded by and sits near the confluence of two rivers offering spectacular views of the mountain peaks and the deep valley.

The *Castle* as it was dubbed is a section of the hotel which is absolutely awesome and conjures a fairy tale experience.

Sara wanted unforgettable memories of her wedding with Raj. She wanted a fabulous experience for all guests who will attend her wedding.

Kailash made all arrangement for her daughter's wedding at the Fairmont. Wedding cards were printed and sent out to more than a hundred of the Nair family members and friends mostly those who lived in the U.S. About 30 guests from Raj's side all of them from India were invited. By the Indian standards, it was a small-sized wedding! Kailash and Sanita were reticent to extend more invitations as the property's charges for food, drink services and the various events planned for the wedding were astronomical.

Sanita was skeptical of her daughter's second nuptial. She still has fond memories of her former son-in-law. He was a gentleman, loved her daughter and caused nothing to hurt her. She wondered how long will Sara's marriage with Raj will last. With the symptoms of ADHD that her daughter is suffering from she wondered, "*Will Raj suffer the same fate as Ash did?*"

The groom's party planned an extravagant procession of *Baraat* with pomp and pageantry. The hotel arranged a carriage which was driven by a single white horse for the groom to ride in accompanied by a live band and singers and dancers from the groom's party to be received by the bride's party. The bride's party did not skimp on expenses and scheduled a variety of Hindu rituals including the *mehndi* ceremony, *sangeeth* musical party and the wedding ceremony, ending with a grand reception.

—

ASH MULLED OVER A PLAN he laid out to take revenge on his ex-wife. The passing of time did not let up his anger for revenge. The more he thought of the stress, hardship and humiliation he endured toward the end of his stay in the U.S. the more determined he became for punishing Sara. His banishment from the U.S. for a decade aggravated him even more. She derailed his meticulously planned strategy to earn his green card and enjoy the freedom to live in the U.S. when he chose to live there and also to live in India.

He purchased a new prepaid phone as planned before and called Victor in America. When Victor answered Ash asked, "Hi Victor, I am now prepared to talk about the mission that I have for you. But before I delve into it, I would like to know your ideas for execution of what I have in mind. Are you okay with this?"

Victor replied, “Sure. What is your planned mission, Ash”?

Ash commenced, “I want my ex-wife punished for what she has done to me. I want to teach her a lesson. I want her to suffer and be scarred psychologically and physically. Let me hear your ideas towards this end goal”.

Victor cleared his voice and said, “I will offer several ways this can be accomplished. However, before we go down that path, let’s talk about what it is going to cost you.”

“Okay. Tell me the cost?” asked Ash.

“Like we discussed the last time we spoke, an investigation of your ex-wife’s present life needs to be conducted. This is important so I can then plan on the actual mission to accomplish. Are you with me?” queried Victor.

“Yes. Tell me what it will cost for the investigation, per se. Then, give me your estimate as a separate line item for completing the mission,” asked Ash.

“Okay. The investigation will involve snooping on her email, listening to her voice conversations over a mobile device and physically tracking her social activities, travel, employment, etc. It also may require getting in touch with the local police informants in Ann Arbor to gather information about her,” elaborated Victor.

Victor stropped for a moment and asked, “Does she use an Android phone?”

Ash replied, “Yes, but that was before the divorce. I bet she still is using her Galaxy as she is reticent to change phones.”

Victor responded, "Okay. Galaxy is easy to listen into and also track her location."

Victor continued, "The investigation will cost you one-hundred thousand dollars, all to be paid up front. I can provide you my bank account and ABA routing numbers so you can wire transfer the money."

Ash asked, "How much does the mission cost?"

Victor replied, "Maiming or otherwise harming the subject will cost one hundred and fifty thousand."

He waited for Ash to react. Ash did not react.

Victor continued, "Murder will cost three hundred grand."

Ash summed up the costs he heard. "So, the investigation and the mission to harm will cost a quarter of a million. The investigation and murder will cost four hundred thousand. Correct?" he asked.

Victor replied, "Yes. That is correct. If you authorize the investigation and the mission, then I suggest you pay me one-half now and the rest upon completion of the job. If you want me to do the investigation now and carry out the mission later, then pay me one hundred now. But don't wait too long after I complete the investigation. I should complete the mission soon after I complete the investigation. Otherwise, the trail may get cold and require a new investigation."

Ash mulled over what Victor said for a few seconds. He responded, "Okay, Victor. Let's do this in phases. Proceed with the phase of investigation first. Start this phases ASAP. Please report to me what you find out about the subject's status and her present activities. Tell me what she is up to now."

Ash wrote down Victor's bank account data on a pad and told him and promised, "You will receive a wire transfer of one hundred thousand from my Fidelity Investments account in a day."

Patience and preparation for Ash' mission are crucial. He waited for the completion of the investigation by Victor before he could commission him to launch the mission.

—

VICTOR GOT TO WORK IMMEDIATELY. He swiftly hacked her laptop and accessed email from her account. Using a special online spy app he was able to geo-locate and track her anonymously whenever she used her phone from the GPS coordinates that her phone revealed. He tapped text messages, photos and calls made and received by her phone.

The target was an easy candidate for Victor to gather information about her present personal life. He met with two local police detectives assigned to the territory where Sara lived to gather any criminal or unethical activities by her. He completed his investigation of Sara in a record time.

The mosaic of data he gathered enabled Victor to stitch together a grand impending plan. The plan he discovered is of her impending destination wedding to Raj at the Fairmont Hotel in Banff. The wedding is scheduled to take place in exactly a week's time.

—

VICTOR GOT ON HIS SMART PHONE and called Ash. With a voice of urgency he said, "Ash, I completed my investigation of your ex-wife. I have important news to report."

Ash asked with great curiosity, "What is it? What did you find out?"

"Your ex-wife is getting married. She is marrying Dr. Raj Kumar. A destination wedding has been planned at the Fairmont Banff Springs Hotel in Banff which is near Calgary in Canada. The wedding is set for exactly a week from today with many events have been planned at the hotel," was the information he dumped.

Ash was in disbelief of what he heard Victor say. He said to himself "*I knew there has always been an ulterior motive behind all the actions Sara took which led to my lockup, despair, humiliation and deportation from America.*"

The anger in him intensified and he renewed his vow to reciprocate the harm she caused to him and then some.

Ash tried to compose himself before he reacted to Victor's report.

Victor interrupted the silence and asked, "Do you have a phase two or a mission in mind for me to carry out? If not, this completes my investigation."

Ash piped up, "Yes, Victor I definitely have a phase two in mind. But I would like to know more about the planned wedding. What information have you gathered about the scheduled wedding? Tell me the details?"

Victor furnished additional details, "Yes, I have a lot of details gathered. The mehndi ceremony is scheduled for the first night of the three-day wedding, followed by a musical party on the second night and then the wedding ceremony on the third day.

"The wedding will end on the same evening with a reception planned in the grand ballroom. All wedding events are planned at the Fairmont hotel. All of the wedding guests have booked their rooms at the hotel also. A special suite has been booked for the bride adjacent to her parents' suite."

Victor added, "By the way, the information I gathered about the wedding also tells that the groom's party planned a gala *Baraat* procession also at the hotel's property on the morning of the wedding ceremony."

Victor stopped and asked, "Would you like to hear more about the wedding?"

Ash replied, "No."

Ash collected his thoughts on the mission he planned. He started to explain, "The mission I have in mind is to have harm done to the bride before her planned wedding. The harm should be carried out swiftly without a prolonged involvement with the subject. We have only a few precious days left to plan and complete it."

Ash paused and continued, "Before I reveal what I have in mind, you are a professional and have experience to carry out a mission like this. Can we talk about the ideas you may have toward this end goal?"

Victor cleared his throat and started to give his strategy, "Ash, I believe in the strategy of the late Chinese military general Sun Tzu. He said something to the effect that the battle is won by choosing the terrain in which it will be fought. Let us establish the terrain for your mission first."

Victor waited for Ash to attentively listen to what he had to say.

He continued, "The terrain should be the Fairmont Hotel. I have been to this property. I intimately know its location and the accommodation and services offered by the hotel staff. It presents the best terrain to wage war. It is a fortuitous coincidence that her wedding is scheduled at a property that I know so well."

Ash responded, "I am okay with the terrain you selected. Please go on."

Victor resumed, "I can slash the bride's carotid artery. I know where this artery is. That severs the trachea. I can do it in a few seconds, I am sure. This requires taking her as hostage. Giving her a sedative like chloroform, put her to sleep and do a fast surgical severance of her carotid artery. I am capable of doing this."

Ash intercepted, "No. I do not want her to be killed, but only harmed. I want her to live and suffer for a prolonged period. I want her to reflect her past and realize the harm she caused to me."

"OK. If those are your objectives, then I suggest I poison her with a pesticide like methyl iodide. I can mix her food with methyl iodide and have her consume it. The consumption will mimic an acute stoke paralyzing her or cause a neuropsychiatric condition. However, the poison may eventually lead to her death. What are her favorite foods?"

"She loves sushi and fond of soups," replied Ash and continued, "Again immediate death is not an option, Victor. She deserves cruel punishment. Do you understand me? Do you have any other ideas?"

Victor offered his second plan of attack, "I can administer a neurotoxin into her body through food. Let me explain what a neurotoxin does. It targets neural components in her body such as her nervous system. The effects are paralysis or weakness in limbs, headache, vision loss, loss of memory and cognitive functions, sexual dysfunction and more. I can name the neurotoxins that are effective, if you like to hear."

Ash responded, "No. Loss of her cognitive function does not appeal to me. I want her mind to continue to work so she can reflect on her past misdeeds."

Victor was beginning to get frustrated with the rejection of his ideas. Nevertheless he continued with his next alternative.

"How about poisoning her using a nerve agent? The Russians have used toxins like organophosphate for poisoning political enemies. I know former KGB officers currently living in the U.S. who can clandestinely procure such toxins from experts in Russia," Victor offered.

Ash remained silent expecting to hear more from Victor.

Victor continued with his suggestion on the use of nerve gas to poison her, "How about deploying novichok? I can have it administered in the form of a spray or ointment. I can bribe the hotel's laundry service to apply novichok to her underwear or I can sneak up into her hotel room and implant it myself. A sure way to administer is to apply the novichok to the inner seams of intimate garments such as a bra or thong where it is retained and will continuously poison her body when the garment is worn. The poison will take three to six hours before she will violently fall ill and go into coma and perish."

"The service staff at the Fairmont is very accommodating. The staff is eager to please their guests and they thrive on the attitude to make everything perfect during their stay. I am sure I can engage the staff to successfully pull off my plan," added Victor.

Ash became uncomfortable with the use of nerve gas. Given the short time left before the wedding Ash felt that clandestinely procuring the nerve agent from the KGB agents may not happen in time. He was uncomfortable with the involvement of the hotel's laundry service or access to her hotel room to implant novichok into her inner clothing. He wondered what if Sara does not use the implanted clothing. Things may go wrong for the sequence of events to take place and succeed.

Ash ruled out Victor's suggestion of nerve gas use. He commented, "Your idea depends on too many variables. It may not work with surety guaranteed, I am afraid."

Victor was getting frustrated at Ash's continued rejections.

Finally he said, "My friend, I have one last plan. That is to create acute radioactive syndrome. I can inject ten micrograms of poisonous polonium-210 isotope into her body. The injection will damage her peripheral nervous system. It will cause a complete hair loss, severe diarrhea and vomiting. She will essentially be paralyzed and will be unable to walk, make her weak, periods of unconsciousness and eventual death."

Victor supplemented, "I can also have this isotope administered through food like sushi which you said she likes."

None of the suggestions Victor made were acceptable to Ash.

Ash conveyed his rejection of them all by generally saying, "Victor, your ideas are good, but none of them will harm her in a flash but seem to take time to inflict injury."

Victor then responded, "Ash, you said you have a plan. Let me hear it, please."

"Yes. I am thinking of an acid attack on her. You are a chemist and what I am about to propose is up your ally. Throw a super acid on her like sulfuric acid, carbonic acid or fluoroantimonic acid?" asked Ash.

Victor listened and waited for Ash to continue.

Ash paused and continued, "Capture her and pour a concentrated super acid on her face and neck. The acid will burn her skin and flesh and disfigure her irreversibly depending on how deep the burning acid penetrates her face and body. Extensive damage to her mouth, throat, nose, eyes and esophagus are possible. She will continue to be alive, be cognitive to think of her past misdeeds, but will be shunned by her would-be new groom and family and friends. That will be a fitting punishment. What do you think? Can you pull this off?"

Victor chimed in, "Yes, of course. It sounds very cut-and-dry. I am a trained chemist and understand what you are saying. I don' think I need to capture her. I can do this in her hotel room. I told you I can get into her hotel room with the help of the hotel service staff who bend over backwards to please their guests."

"However, let me propose a modification to your proposal," said Victor

"What is it?" inquisitively asked Ash.

"After I capture her in her room, I should sedate her by using chloroform or another quick acting sedative. After she is fully sedated, throw the acid on her. If she is not sedated, she may scream when the acid singes her skin and flesh which may immediately draw the attention of other guests and hotel staff. She may also rush into the bathroom and wash off the acid, which defeats the mission," was Victor's detailed reply.

Ash responded, "I am okay with your modification."

"Victor, tell me this. Can you get hold of the acid in Canada? These acids may be controlled substances there?" queried Ash.

Victor quickly replied, "No problem. I can easily get hold of concentrated sulfuric acid in Calgary. The acid is clear and sold in convenient and transparent bottles. Smuggling the bottles into the hotel is going to be easy."

"Ash, if you do not have further question, this sounds like a plan. It is simple and straight forward. I am prepared to execute it. I will determine the right day and time for its execution. I will try to have the attack carried out before the wedding ceremony. Okay?" asked Victor.

While waiting for Ash's reply Victor asked, "Do you really want to this, Ash? The acid will permanently disfigure her."

Ash emphatically replied, "Yes."

Before switching off his phone, Victor reminded, "Ash, remember my fees that we talked about previously? You should send me half of the fee I quoted for the mission. Please wire it to me - same account number."

Ash wanted Victor to confirm the fee they discussed, "Seventy-five thousand dollars, correct?"

Victor replied, "That is correct."

Ash's final statement, "You will see this payment in your account by tomorrow."

—

It was Tuesday evening in Hyderabad. Sara's second wedding is scheduled to take place in less than four days in Canada. Ash sat with his parents for a delicious south Indian dinner that his mother prepared with curried prawns served on basmati rice as the main course. Ash did not share with his parents his secret plot against his ex-wife.

As a concerned mother looking after the wellbeing of her children Rupa brought up the subject of Ash to remarry. She opened with, "Ash, you have been divorced for nearly seven months. You have a good job now with CVS working from home. Are you ready to look at a potential partner to marry again?"

Ash replied, "No, Mom I am not."

He waited a long minute and spoke again, "I am still angry and deeply saddened by my failed marriage with Sara."

Ash then felt compelled to report, "I heard that Sara is getting married again."

The parents Rupa and Sunil suddenly became curious. They asked a bevy of questions, "Who, when, where, how did you find out about her marriage?"

Without revealing that he obtained this information through hired investigators in the U.S. and in India Ash detailed Sara's past romantic relationship with Raj when they were in the med school in Osmania.

Dinner was done, but the conversation they started was not. They sat in their comfortable cushioned furniture in the living room with tumblers of iced water on the cocktail table in front of them. The ceiling fan was whirring quietly and kept the room cool.

Rupa commenced, "You and Sara had a failed relationship in your marriage whether it was because of her or you or a combination of both."

Sunil expressed his regret, "I wish I had a background check done on Sara before we fixed her matrimony with you. That may have revealed her relationship with Raj and you may have rejected her as your partner."

Rupa continued to advise her son about his ex-wife. She said, "Ash let her be. Sara found her old flame with who she romanticized before settling for you. She's out of your life now. Luckily, you do not have any alimony or child-support obligations to her, which is a silver lining that I see."

Ash protested still seething in anger, "Mom, Sara needs to be punished for harming me. Would a sane person report to the Secret Service that I threatened to kill the president of the United States? She should be taught a lesson." He blurted in a fit of passion.

Rupa responded in a calm voice, "Teaching a lesson to another human being, no less your former wife with whom you shared intimate relationship for years, is not for you. Only God will punish those who sinned, my son."

Rupa paused for a while and posed this query, "Ash, do you remember the Hindu virtue of ahimsa?"

Ash replied, "Only vaguely. I know what ahimsa generally means which is not cause harm to others," expecting his mother to explain the details.

Rupa explained, "Ahimsa is nonviolence. It applies to all living beings. It is total avoidance of harming of any kind of living creatures, not only by deeds, but also by words and thoughts."

Rupa ventured to give an example of ahimsa in real life, "Do you know about the founder of modern independent India, Mahatma Gandhi? He believed in and practiced ahimsa."

She elaborated, “Before the turn of the previous century, Gandhi was a practicing barrister in South Africa. He was publicly humiliated when he was traveling by train from Pretoria. He was seated in a first-class compartment when a white man complained of a brown-skinned man sharing space with him. A white train conductor told him that coolies were not allowed in the first-class compartment. Gandhi resisted, producing his ticket and refusing to budge. He was forcibly pushed out of the train in to the cold, rugged outdoors.”

Rupa continued, “That incident of discrimination was a transformative event in Gandhi’s life. He launched a movement of nonviolence against the British, who were ruling South Africa then.”

She continued the example of ahimsa, “Later Gandhi returned to India and applied his nonviolent resistance against the British who were also ruling India then. He endured several long jail sentences in South Africa and India, forced by the British.”

“Ultimately, through his nonviolent protests and belief in ahimsa Gandhi was able to free India from the tyranny of the British who ruled our country for over two centuries and plundered our country’s resources and made the Indians subservient to the British Monarchy,” Rupa concluded.

Sunil chimed in by saying, “No shots were fired by the Indians and no harm was done to the British despite the harm to Gandhi’s personal ego, public humiliation, jail sentences and damage to his reputation as a barrister and open discrimination against Indians. Although the British soldiers massacred thousands of Gandhi’s followers of his nonviolence movement, his tolerance for hate and belief in ahimsa saved the lives of millions of other people. At the end, Gandhi achieved the result he desired."

—

Ash's life was becoming easy and comfortable in Hyderabad surrounded by his old friends and relatives.

The discussion of the spiritual doctrine of ahimsa with his parents had a profound impact on Ash. The explanation by his parents of this spiritual principle demonstrated how it works and led Ash to certain conviction. It was uplifting. He was reawakened into knowing the difference from right and wrong. He was beginning to come to his senses.

He kept mulling over and over again the discussion he had with his parents. He said to him, "*I am grateful for my loving and well-informed parents. I am grateful for all of the blessings in my life. I must do what is right now.*"

It began to dawn upon Ash that the mission he commissioned Victor to undertake to harm his ex-wife is not right.

CHAPTER

14

IT IS FOUR DAYS BEFORE Sara's destination wedding at the Fairmont Banff Springs Hotel in early June. Sara booked her flight and made land arrangements in Calgary to arrive at the hotel four days before her planned wedding. That allowed a full night and a day to relax at the hotel before the first event of mehndi commenced.

Her parents and younger brother left three days earlier. Her parents went early to check on the wedding arrangements at the hotel that they made and orchestrate the details to perfection.

Sara exchanged email with Raj. He and his entourage of relatives and friends traveled from India and already arrived in Calgary and checked in to the Fairmont.

Sara packed her suitcases with a variety of special Indian outfits to wear at the wedding. They included designer Indian wedding dresses, *lehenga* choli attire, *salwar kameez* dresses, a variety of formal saree ensembles, and an interesting collection of Bollywood dresses that she planned to use at various wedding events. She packed more clothes than she needed to wear at her wedding.

In her large Gucci handbag she packed a dozen sets of jewelry for wearing at the wedding. The jewelry was custom designed bridal jewelry and made from highly refined twenty four carat gold and authentic natural diamonds, natural pearls and other precious cut stones. The jewelry was intended to perfectly match with the dresses or other garments she will wear. Some jewelry sets composed of a necklace, ear hangings and nose piece were neatly encased in special ultra-thin boxes. She inserted the others in small silk pouches. Sara neatly tucked the boxes and pouches in her handbag. Her handbag alone seemed to weigh more than fifteen pounds.

A last minute change detained Sara at home. Her girlfriends from Pioneer High and University of Michigan wanted to throw a bachelorette party for her in Ann Arbor. Sara felt obligated to attend the party even though it was scheduled for the day of her planned departure to Banff.

She rebooked her flight to travel on the day as her mehndi event. The flight was scheduled to depart Detroit International Airport at 8:30 AM and arrive in Calgary International at 12:30 PM. She figured that with a two-hour car ride from Calgary she would be at the Fairmont in Banff around 3 PM. Mehndi was scheduled for 6 that evening.

—

THE PARTY WAS AT DIAMONDBACK Saloon in Ann Arbor. Sara is no longer a prolific drinker, but at the bachelorette party she succumbed to the pressure of her friends to drink. A live band played country music and people got out on the large dance floor and did line dancing. Some did the 2-step.

"You gals forced me to cancel my spa appointment that was scheduled for this evening at the Fairmont Hotel by arranging this party. I wanted to get rejuvenated at the spa before my wedding," said Sara by looking at her girlfriends.

One of her girlfriends replied, "Sara, don't worry. I am sure you can get your spa treatment at the Fairmont after you get there. You will have plenty of time to relax and pretty up for your first night with your new husband."

Many guys hung around the large bar at the Saloon. Sara was having fun with her friends reminiscing of her good old days.

At one point an announcer asked, "Are there any women whose boy friends were out hunting? If they are alone, they should all bring up one dollar to the bar for some 'buck shots'. No limit on drinks."

Sara's friends took up on that offer and bought the announced drinks. Sara ended up drinking half a dozen buck shots while chatting with them and the guys at the bar and had a wonderful time.

—

When her friends dropped her off at her house it was past 2 AM. Sara tried to sleep. She got four hours and awakened by the sound of her alarm clock. The Uber driver arrived 7 AM and drove her to the airport in Detroit.

She checked in her suitcases and carried her large and heavy bag of jewelry in her arm. She was bleary eyed and half-drunk as she boarded the Delta flight to Calgary. She slept on the plane. Several cups of black coffee she drank on the plane did not seem to fully wake her up as she left the plane at the Calgary airport.

The flight arrived fifteen minutes early in Calgary. She felt good that she has ample time to drive the eighty miles of distance and arrive at the hotel on time. She rented a Toyota Prius at the airport. This hybrid is her favorite car to drive as it is quiet and enabled to hear better when she took calls on her mobile phone; roomy inside and easy to drive. She specifically asked for a red Prius when she made the reservation with the rental car company since she believed red brings good luck to her new marriage. She got a black Prius, instead.

The navigation system in the Prius guided her to travel west on Trans Continental Highway #1 toward Banff. As she got on the four-lane divided highway she noticed a white on green-maple leaf route sign posted with the words Trans-Canada Hwy. She looked at her watch. It was two O' clock in the afternoon. As she headed west, the open fields slid endlessly away under a clear blue sky.

—

JEREMIAH JONES IS A lumberjack from the Seattle area. He is twenty-two years old and had a high school diploma. He loved being independent and care free. He had a stable, persistent and thrifty personality. He loved the outdoors and working in isolated areas like the woods. Something about the fragrance of freshly cut trees appealed to him.

He started his job in the logging industry because the pay was good. He had a learner's permit and received on-the-job training to become familiar with the forest environment and learn how to operate logging machinery. He received training in all aspect of the logging industry. He was trained as a faller to cut down tall trees in the forest, as a logging equipment operator to sheer the limbs of the fallen trees and cut them into desired lengths and as a logging truck operator to drag the denuded logs to the deck and transport them to the mills for ultimate processing into forest products by the industry and ultimately for use by the consumer.

Jeremiah was conscientious and knew the demands and dangers of his job. After he qualified as a logging truck driver he settled into the job of transporting logs from the forest to the mill by driving the logging trucks owned by the Latten Trucking, Inc. He loved being an independent contractor and set his own timetable for the days and hours to work. The money he earned dictated his hours. He typically made two thousand dollars per week completing fifteen runs per week between the log's loading areas in the forest to the processing mill.

Jeremiah was aware of the accidents involving logging trucks with smaller passenger vehicles due to improper loading, speeding, unsafe roads, defective and damaged reflectors on the truck, improper maintenance of trucks by the trucking company.

He was aware that sometimes logs fall from the loader. A thousand pound log falling on a passenger vehicle will smash the vehicle and cause instant death to the passengers riding in it. Luckily he had not been involved in an accident while driving a logging truck.

It was 1:30 PM on a normal weekday. Jeremiah just completed eating the turkey sandwich and a bag of potato chips he brought in his lunch box. He finished drinking a can of diet coke. He was ready to go.

The sky was blue and the air was crisp and cool in early summer.

He started the day at seven in the morning and drove an hour from his trailer home to the trucking company's loader. He already made two runs between the loader and the mill and delivered more than a hundred and fifty logs. This was his third run for the day and the last. He wanted to call it a day after he returned the truck to the forest. He was getting tired and looked forward to going home.

Like he did on his two runs earlier in the day, Jeremiah had his logging truck loaded with hundred foot long logs with eighty logs piled up into neat rows one row on top of another. He attached the logs from the front to the rear end of the truck using heavy chains. He attached a three foot long metal chain to a wire that passed over the top of the load. In addition he used straps to hold the logs tightly in place as an extra precaution from accidentally falling off the truck.

The internal scale built into the truck registered a weight of a shade below forty tons, which is below the weight limit on the roads.

Jeremiah set out on a twelve percent grade of the logging gravel road and slowly made a right turn to the main road that ran parallel to the highway to ultimately join the Trans Canadian Highway #1.

Jeremiah carefully maneuvered his logging truck on to the highway joining the stream of local traffic of passenger cars, vans, RV's, trucks with attached trailers and fuel trucks. The truck was capable of use on rough ground and hilly trails in the forest as well as transport on a normal highway. It was designed to provide low ground pressure and good traction even on wet roads which Jeremiah liked.

Jeremiah enjoyed the scenery of majestic Rocky Mountains and green meadows as he kept his eyes on the traffic directly ahead on the traffic behind as reflected in his rear view and side view mirrors. Everything appeared normal. He drove at a steady clip of sixty miles per hour, as he normally did under similar road and weather conditions. The processing mill is only fifteen miles away where he will off load the logs his truck was hauling.

—

SARA IS SCHEDULED to be at the Fairmont Hotel at 3 PM. It was already two O' clock on her watch. A highway sign that she just passed read that Banff is seventy miles ahead. Sara was getting impatient that she is stuck behind a logging truck. She was unable to move over to the left lane and pass the log truck as traffic was heavy and she could not quickly make her move.

Sara was impatient to be stuck behind the logging truck with piled up logs on it. She already trailed the truck for the last couple of miles unable to pass it. She was getting restless without a clear view of the road ahead as the logging truck with its tall stacked up load totally obstructed her view.

She decided to pass the logging truck which was speeding down a hilly part of the highway. It meant she needed to quickly veer the Prius into the fast moving lane on her left, accelerate to pass the truck on her right and after passing return to the right lane when the truck is at a safe distance behind the Prius. Her adrenaline flowed at the maneuver she was about to make.

Just then her mobile phone rang. She decided hold off on her planned maneuver to overtake the truck. She stayed back in her lane. She grabbed the ringing phone that lay on the car's seat next to her. She grabbed the phone using her right hand and checked the screen. The caller was Raj. She swiped it using her right thumb. As she swiped the phone it slipped and fell to her feet. Without thinking she instinctively leaned down to pick up the dropped phone. While picking up the phone her right foot which was on the gas pedal unexpectedly pushed the pedal suddenly accelerating the Prius.

Just then Jeremiah who was driving the logging truck in her front also slowed down.

"BAAM!"

The Prius rear ended the logging truck.

There were violent bumps and crunches followed by horrid scraping and ripping sound.

The Prius penetrated the rear bumper of the truck. The airbag in the Prius was immediately activated.

The force of the collision rattled the straps and chains that Jeremiah used to bind the heavy logs on his truck. Jeremiah heard the loud sound that came from the rear of his truck. He realized something hit his truck from the back. He immediately activated the air brakes in his truck to bring it to a sudden stop.

The sudden deceleration of the logging truck added momentum to the logs which already started their motion toward the Prius.

"SWOOSH", "BANG".

Logs from the truck started to slide toward its back.

The Prius was impaled by five logs from the front windshield to the back window. The Prius came to a screeching halt butting against the truck

Because Sara was not in the upright position in her seat she was not crushed by the penetrating logs, but when she raised her head two more logs from the truck whumped and fiercely penetrated a gap in the broken windshield above the steering wheel. One log smashed against Sara's right side of her face. She turned her head away to avoid the log. A second log slammed into the left side of her face. Before she knew what happened, her head and face ended up in a tight gap between the two new impaled logs. The moving logs sheared her face violently from both sides causing major physical injuries.

Her eyes, nose and cheeks burned. She opened her eyes with difficulty and she saw little. Everything was white and out of focus. Her blurred vision filled with tears flowing like a flood down her cheeks.

Her head was spinning. She felt blood dripping from her forehead and nose. She felt the long, sharp and rough splinters from the logs skewered her face and neck and the upper part of her chest.

She noticed that new logs from the truck continued to tumble on the Prius and pile up atop it crushing the roof of the vehicle. The roof was severely distorted, but the impaled logs prevented it from making contact with Sara's head and also prevented injury to her brain.

Sara's head squeezed between the heavy and abrasive logs compressed her ears. She thought that her ear drums collapsed. She could not hear a sound. She wanted to throw up, but couldn't as her head was lodged between the logs. She controlled her vomiting.

She tried to move her toes inside the soft shoes she wore. She couldn't. She tried to move her fingers. Again, no sensation and she couldn't move them.

Sara thought this was her last living moment. She screamed out loud, but did not hear her own scream. She cried out in agony.

"I am going to die. God, I don't want to die. Not now," she prayed.

"I don't want to die . . . God . . . please no. NO," she cried

"Please. God forgive me for whatever I have done," her voice repented loudly.

—

EMERGENCY SERVICES OF FIREMEN, ambulance and a priest arrived within five minutes at the scene of the crash. The firemen assessed the scene before the paramedics could render emergency medical assistance to the passengers in the car. They did not know how many passengers were inside as the pile of logs completely obstructed their view of the interior of the car.

The wreckage reeked of gasoline spilled from the Prius when the heavy load of the fallen logs ruptured its fuel tank. The firemen manually rolled out the logs that were piled on the top of the car one-by-one before getting to the logs that impaled the vehicle. They noticed seven logs penetrated the car from the front windshield to the back and a bloodied passenger was lodged between two of those logs.

The firemen got to work as they were dealing with a life-threatening situation. With chainsaws the firemen cut through five of the logs that penetrated and were lodged in the car, leaving untouched the two logs that wedged the passenger in the driver's seat. They smashed out what is left of the window glass in the doors of the car and gently pushed out the portions of the log that they were unable to cut from the outside because they were lodged inside the vehicle.

The firemen exercised extreme care while cutting to ensure that no sparks were produced which could ignite the spilled fuel on the ground.

The firemen now had a better view of the occupants in the vehicle. They assessed that no other passengers were inside the vehicle. They noticed severe bleeding from the skull, face and neck of the passenger.

They assessed the situation. The only way they could avoid disturbing the passenger without causing her further injury is by vehicle extrication.

They summoned the Jaws of Life equipment. This was the only solution left to safely initiate the complicated extrication of the vehicle.

More than an hour elapsed since the crash. The passenger is severely injured and is in pain. Urgent paramedic assistance is needed, but they cannot extricate the injured until she is freed up from the logs that were wedging her head, neck and upper body.

The operator of the Jaws of Life equipment decided that a full roof removal is what is needed. He first anchored the Prius to the road so it would not move as he used the Jaws of Life equipment and cause further injury and pain to the passenger.

He carefully cut the forward roof flap. Then the roof was folded backwards providing access to the logs from the top. The operator pulled out the jammed driver's door as well as the passenger's door. He carefully rolled out the logs that wedged the passenger so her head is freed up for extrication. When the logs were rolled out the passenger's head suddenly slumped toward her chest and she became unconscious.

The firefighters returned to action. They removed the steering wheel by slicing with a mini cutter to prevent leg injury or posterior dislocation of the hip. After the seat belt was cut, the paramedics took over the scene.

By carefully sliding their hands underneath the spine of the passenger the paramedics rapidly extricated Sara from the wrecked car. He was placed on a stretcher. Immediate first aid was quickly administered by the paramedics. A hospital helicopter bearing a Red Cross sign that hovered above the accident scene picked the injured passenger and whisked her to the Foothills Medical Center in Calgary.

After Sara was evacuated from the damaged Prius a firefighter returned to inspect the contents left inside the car before towing it away for forensic analysis. He noticed Sara's large Gucci bag which spilled out pieces of brilliant gold and sparkling diamond jewelry. The individual diamonds that Sara packed in her bag got dislodged from their intricate settings into beautiful necklaces and were strewn on the floor of the car. The firefighter picked up the sparkling diamonds piece by piece and inserted them back into a necklace box for later delivery to Sara at the hospital.

The necklace box in which the firefighter reinserted the loose diamonds had this written inside, "To: Sara. Best Thanksgiving Day Ever! With Love and Affection! From: Sunil & Rupa Sharma."

—

Sara was rushed into the trauma operating room where surgical operations were carried out by trauma-trained surgeons and nurses. She was placed in an aseptic environment of the intensive care unit and was induced into a coma by administering drugs. Hours of observation and testing by many medical specialists found that the physical injuries she suffered were extensive. She suffered a major injury to her spinal cord causing paralysis of her body from the neck down. She suffered damage to her head, neck, eyes, nose, mouth including her teeth structure, and ears, facial bone structure damage, and pierced soft tissue in her chest.

—

SARA'S PARENTS RUSHED to the Medical Center when they found about it as they were getting set up for the mehndi ceremony at the hotel. Raj joined to see his bride. It was past six O'clock in the evening when they reached the hospital.

Because of the extent of the injury and her lock up in the ICU sedated by drugs, they were denied a personal visitation to see her up close and speak with her. They had to settle for a look from a distance through a glass partition. The only thing they could see was Sara lying on a hospital bed sedated and hooked up to machines whose beeps they could hear. Her head and face were fully wrapped with white bandages.

The attending physician at the ICU took them to the meditation room at the Center. He spoke with a soft tone. Addressing Kailash, who he knew is the patient's father, the physician said "You should be thankful that your daughter is alive after the horrific accident she had this afternoon. She suffered extensive trauma and physical injuries that we were able to diagnose so far."

The doctor tried to be optimistic. He continued, "We have the best doctors and state-of-the-art technology and equipment here at the FMC. I am confident that we can put her body together, but it will take time."

Raj asked, "How long will it take for her to recover?" reminding the doctor that her wedding was planned in a couple of days.

The doctor sympathetically replied, "I am so sorry to hear about her impending wedding. Unfortunately, it will be months, if not years before the physical injuries can be corrected and heal. The trauma she experienced will last a lot longer to recover from."

The doctors waited for what he told Raj to sink in. He asked, "Are you the groom?"

Raj responded with tears in his eyes, "Yes."

The physician glumly added, "She suffered a spinal cord injury. She does not show sensation in her fingers and toes. We could not detect sensation in her arms and legs, either. She suffers from paralysis of her body from nick down. I am sorry!"

—

VICTOR WHO ARRIVED in Banff the day before Sara's arrival has been monitoring Sara's movements by tracking her phone and recording her email and text messages. He knew about the car wreck she was involved in. Actually he heard the "BAAM" sound when her Prius collided with the logging truck through her smart phone which she activated before the accident to answer the call received from Raj. Victor had a recording of Sara's groans and her appeal to God after the crash because of her activated phone.

He read a full description of Sara's injuries by reading the e-Paper of Calgary Herald and from Calgary Sun.

Victor wanted to gather more information about the extent of Sara's injuries before calling Ash the day after the accident.

—

Ash had an awakening to the Hindu spiritual doctrine of ahimsa after his parents enlightened him with. He was beginning to seriously think over what they advised about leaving Sara to live her life.

"Harming Sara who he loved once is not ethical or moral", he convinced himself.

It dawned on Ash that the concepts of revenge of an eye-for-an-eye and a tooth-for-a-tooth are mostly Western concepts. Now that Ash is immersed back in the Hindu religion and culture his thoughts on revenge simmered down.

With the words of advice he received from his older brother to close the chapter on his ex-wife; and more recently the advice and wisdom from his mother, Ash completely rethought his pursuit of revenge against his ex-wife.

He decided to call Victor and pull the plug on the cruel mission against Sara that he commissioned him to carry out.

It was evening in Hyderabad and a new day was dawning in the Canadian Rockies. As before, using a purchased prepaid old phone, Ash called Victor.

It was seven in the morning for Victor. He was awakened by the ringing phone.

Victor answered the phone and groggily said, "Yes."

Before Ash could say a word, recognizing it was Ash on the other end, Victor exclaimed, "Mission accomplished!"

Ash's heart raced and his emotions suddenly peaked. With adrenaline pumping he bombarded him with a series of rapid questions,

"What? Where are you? Did you already go through with the mission? Was Sara harmed?"

Victor replied, "I am in Banff where your ex-wife's wedding is scheduled to take place tomorrow morning."

Victor paused and continued, "No, I did not have to pull off any mission, Ash."

He calmly added, "God fulfilled the mission."

Victor then played a recording of Sara's repent to God as she lay crushed in her car seat after the logs hit her body, "Please. God forgive me for whatever I have done."

Ash was stunned to silence.

Victor then provided the gory details of how the accident happened and how Sara was trapped for hours before she was extricated from the car and rushed to the hospital. He relayed the news of the extensive physical and traumatic injuries she received as reported in the Calgary newspapers.

Ash did not have anything further to say after listening to Victor's detailed narration of the unfortunate and tragic accident and its aftermath except a thought that popped into his head. He waited for a long minute before speaking.

"Victor, I am so glad that you did not bring about this tragedy to my ex-wife," he said with compassion.

Ash saw a silver lining in this horrible tragedy which he wished did not take place at all. He said to himself: "*God is mysterious. God handled in His own Devine way a fitting retribution for the suffering I endured because of Sara's wanton and willful acts to unfairly punish me.*"

Ash collected this thoughts and finally said, "Victor, yes. The mission has been accomplished! I agree."

Ash murmured under his breath, "Sara is now locked up in her fortress of solitude."

Victor did not hear Ash's inaudible final words as he already switched off his mobile device.

ABOUT THE AUTHOR

T.R. COCA

The author has a rare combination of multi-disciplined education, a kaleidoscopic professional career and rich cultural background. His first love of Physics drove him to the pinnacle of leaning of Physics, as evidenced by the degrees he earned which are B.S., M.S., M. A., and Ph.D. While working as a Physics teacher and later as a Physicist at General Dynamics Corporation, TR pursued law to earn his J.D. and synergistically combined his scientific background with knowledge of the law and became an U.S. Intellectual Property attorney. TR has been admitted to practice in New York, Ohio, Vermont and the United States Patent Bar. He is admitted to practice before Court of Appeals for the Federal Circuit and the Supreme Court of the United States.

Before serving as the Vice President and Chief Intellectual Property Law Counsel at International Game Technology Corp. He championed patent litigation and licensing as a Senior Director at NVIDIA Corporation. Prior to that, TR spearheaded as a Corporate IP Counsel at IBM for over two decades. At IBM he orchestrated many Executive and Senior management positions in many world locations including a five-year international assignment as the Assistant General Counsel in charge of IP in IBM's Asia Pacific Headquarters in Tokyo. Prior to IBM, he capitalized as a Patent Lawyer at NCR Corporation and as a Senior Research Engineer at General Dynamics Corp.

Of Indian heritage, TR has gainfully combined his rich and disciplined Indian cultural upbringing with the consensus building of the Japanese tradition that he was exposed to while living in Japan and the competitive and innovative work ethic prevalent in the United States.

TR presented and published over fifty papers and talks on Physics, intellectual property, and corporate law matters, including contributing a chapter on the Semiconductor Chip Protection Law to the legal treatise *Intellectual Property Litigation & Licensing*. He served for three years on the Editorial Board of the *AIPLA Quarterly Journal* of the American Intellectual Property Law Association. In April 2020 he chronicled his life in the title *The Green Card Dowry Plan* published by Ingram Spark. He published his second book titled *Heptagon Writings* in October 2020, which is a collection of essays, published also by Ingram Spark.

T.R.'s kaleidoscopic work experience has been as a physics teacher, physicist, software architect, intellectual property attorney, litigator, mentor, editor, public speaker, and writer.

www.ingramcontent.com/pod-product-compliance
Lightning Source LLC
Chambersburg PA
CBHW021059080526
44587CB00010B/300
* 9 7 8 1 7 3 4 5 3 3 8 5 9 *

Ang Saligan ng Pananampalataya

PAGLALAKBAY PATUNGO SA HARI!

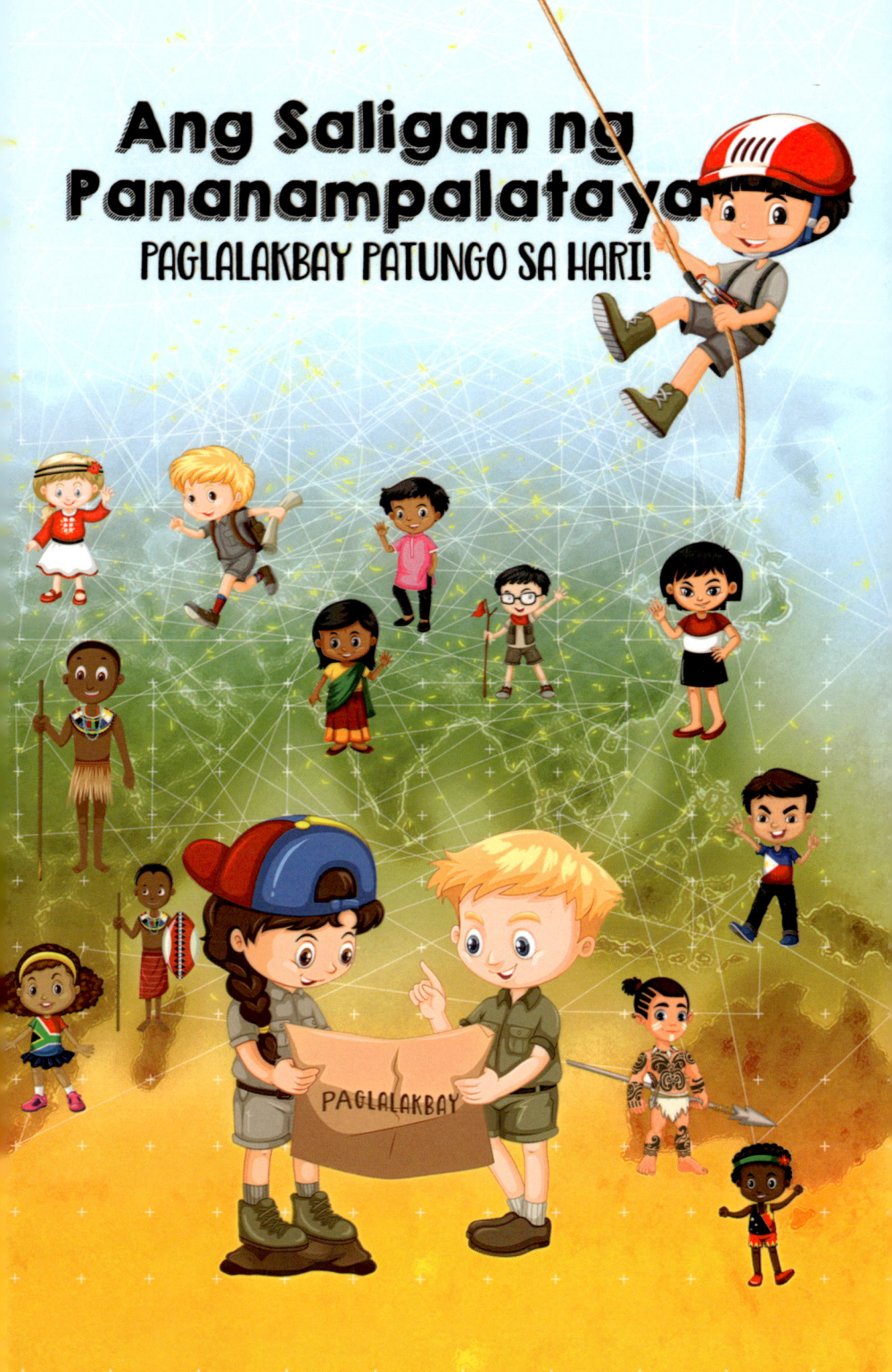

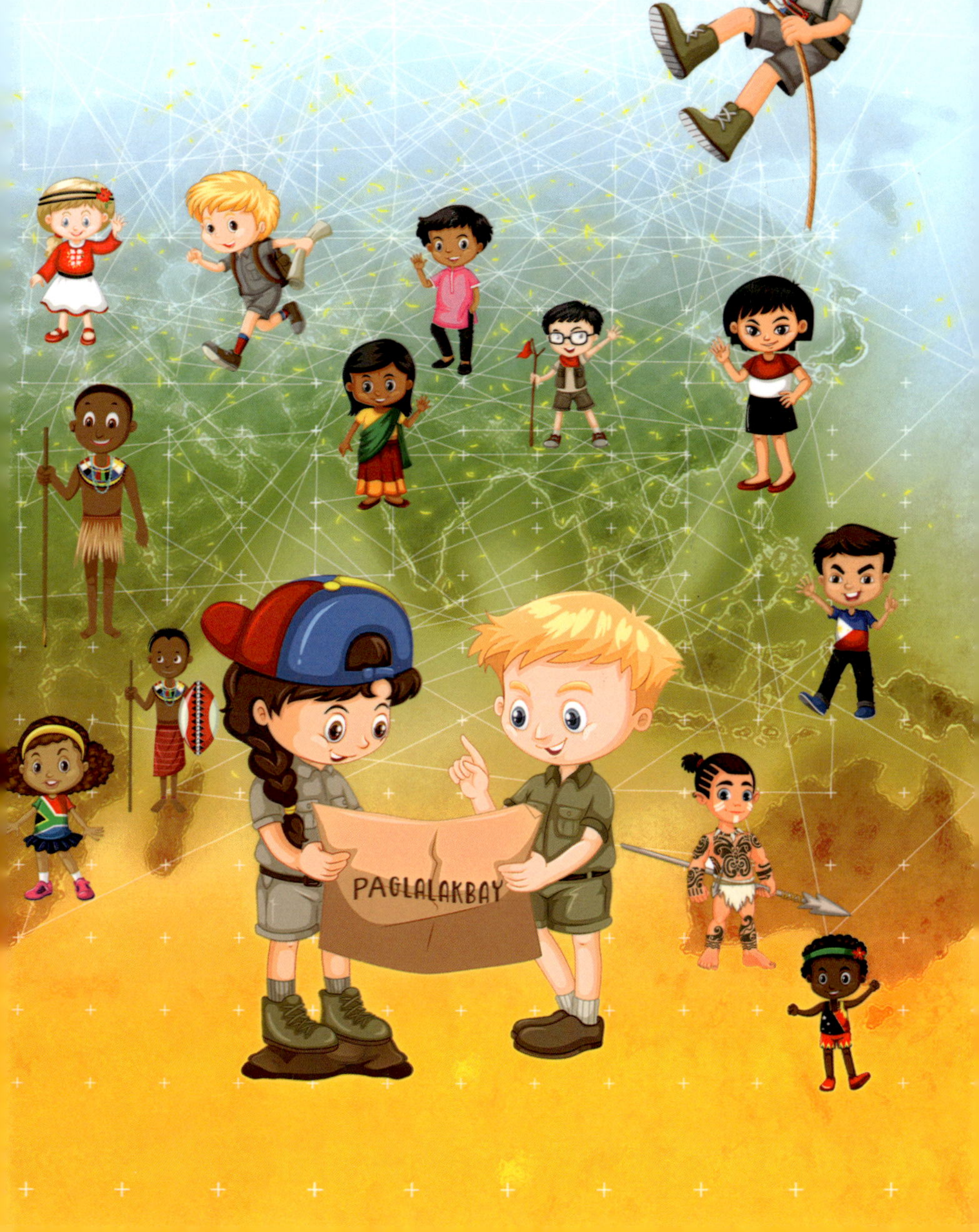